Redeeming Our Cracks

Redeeming Our Cracks

Prayers, poems, reflections and stories
on mental health and well-being

Neil Paynter (Ed)

wild goose
publications

www.**ionabooks**.com

Contents of book © individual contributors
Compilation © 2023 Neil Paynter

First published 2023 by
Wild Goose Publications
Suite 9, Fairfield, 1048 Govan Road, Glasgow G51 4XS, Scotland
the publishing division of the Iona Community.
Scottish Charity No. SC003794. Limited Company Reg. No. SC096243.

ISBN 978-1-80432-265-9

Cover image © Shekakaka | Dreamstime.com

The publishers gratefully acknowledge the support of the Drummond Trust, 3 Pitt Terrace, Stirling FK8 2EY in producing this book.

All rights reserved. Apart from the circumstances described below relating to non-commercial use, no part of this publication may be reproduced in any form or by any means, including photocopying or any information storage or retrieval system, without written permission from the publisher via PLSclear.com.

Non-commercial use:
The material in this book may be used non-commercially for worship and group work without written permission from the publisher. If photocopies of sections are made, please make full acknowledgement of the source, and report usage to CLA or other copyright organisation.

Neil Paynter has asserted his right in accordance with the Copyright, Designs and Patents Act, 1988, to be identified as the author of this compilation
and the individual contributors have asserted their rights to be identified as authors of their contributions.

Overseas distribution
Australia: Willow Connection Pty Ltd, 1/13 Kell Mather Drive, Lennox Head, NSW 2478
New Zealand: Pleroma, Higginson Street, Otane 4170, Central Hawkes Bay

Printed in the UK by Page Bros (Norwich) Ltd

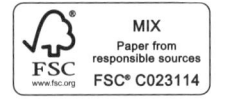

Contents

Introduction 11

PRAYERS

Surprises and gifts 14

Cactus, Sandra Sears 14
Surprising gifts, Jean Hudson 14
On mundane days, Janet Lees 15
Big Bang theory, Sandra Sears 16
Fragments, Sandra Sears 16
Still small voice, Elizabeth Baxter 17

Community 18

Swallows, Jean Hudson 18
A lineup for the exhausted, Janet Lees 19
A prayer for real church, Simon Taylor 19
Alyas' prayer, Alyas 20
At times like this, Janet Lees 21
Dove of Peace, Simon Taylor 22
Calling disciples, Janet Lees 22
Breath prayer, Elizabeth Baxter 23
Rising Christa, Elizabeth Baxter 24

Prayers of concern 25

Prayer for all with invisible illnesses, John Butterfield 25
God of healing and wholeness (based on Psalm 116:5), Kathy Crawford 25
A prayer for those who offer pastoral care, Simon Taylor 27
God of community, Elizabeth Baxter 28
Prayer for ourselves, Elizabeth Baxter 30

Darkness and light 31

The evening draws on, Elizabeth Baxter 31
The night draws in, Elizabeth Baxter 31
Dying darkness, Sandra Sears 31
Calling One (A psalm), Janet Lees 32
Prayer from a prayer-writing workshop at Dove Café, Susan Palmer 33

Healing prayer, John Butterfield   34
Scars, Sandra Sears   34
Still praying, Janet Lees   36
An Easter prayer, Elizabeth Baxter   36
Like the catkins, Jean Hudson   37
Dance of life, Elizabeth Baxter   38
Still calling, Janet Lees   39
Prayer of re-turn, Bev Robertson   39
Journeying prayer, Elizabeth Baxter   40
Phos Hilaron (O gracious Light!), Jessica Wachter   40

Prayers of thanksgiving and praise   42

Every day, Susan Palmer   42
In emotional turmoil, Pamela Turner   42
Beginning to emerge from bereavement, Katy Owen   43
Thank you for old friends, Neil Paynter   43
A psalm of thanksgiving, Neil Paynter   44
Examine me, Janet Lees   44

Prayers for protection, safety, comfort and rest   46

Prayer for protection, Elizabeth Baxter   46
A safe place, Simon Taylor   47
We come, Holy One, Kathy Swaar   48
God's cushions, Janet Lees   50
Angel of the North, Pamela Turner   50
The promise, Jean Hudson   51
Soothe me, Lord, Ann Jepson   52
The answer, David Norman   52
Holy Spirit, Emma Major   53

Blessings   54

A blessing for those who are depressed, Neil Paynter   54
Blessing for a carer, Kathy Crawford   54
A blessing for those who have no one left to talk to, Neil Paynter   55
Bless us, Ruth Burgess   56
Give me a smile, Ruth Burgess   56
When, Ruth Burgess   57
Along roads and byways, Ruth Burgess   57

REDEEMING OUR CRACKS: A LITURGY ON CHANGING PERSPECTIVES ON MENTAL ILL HEALTH, Yvonne Morland   59

POEMS

Write bravely, poems by Emma Major   66

Depression   66
I wear a mask   67
Can you see me?   67
Grey days   68
Rock-bottom dumps   69
Courage   69
Gentle winds   70
Wisdom   71
Know my peace   71
Eye of the storm   72
Anxiety   72
Me, myself and I   73
Surviving in the dark   74
Write bravely   75
Peace descends   75

Pilgrimage, poems by Rosie Miles   76

You come here   76
Good Friday   77
My sadness   78
Wound   78
May your brow be blessed   78
Pilgrimage   78
Bethesda   79

Finding the fish, poems by Christine Dowling   80

Tribute to M   80
I'm losing my mum to dementia   81
You see love on the dementia ward   82
Finding the fish   83

8   Redeeming our cracks

The day I lost my mum, poems by Tricia Creamer   84

The day I lost my Mum   84
Family confusion   84
The week my mother lay dying   85
Clearing the papers   86

What is happiness?, poems by Janet Lees   88

One of those days   88
What is happiness?   88
Lost   90
All cracked up (In Ampleforth Abbey)   90
With arms open   91

Bipolar story, poems by David Norman   93

Meditation on the Trinity   94
Bipolar story   95
Love   97
The rocky boat   97
Found   98

Craftswoman, poems by Bev Robertson   100

The lost message   100
Craftswoman   101

Some more poems   102

Homage to young men, Alastair McIntosh   102
Receiving (A poem for John), Rachel McCann   104
A poem by Glyn, Glyn   106
Depression, Linda Hill   106
Names matter, Simon Taylor   110
Gerry, Neil Paynter   111
Anathema, Pamela Turner   114
It was easy for you, John Butterfield   115
When I have lost my song (Matt 6:25–34), Elizabeth Baxter   116
The hollow, Robert Shooter   116
Under the comet, Peter Charles Jackson   118
Myself, Warren Bardsley   120

Watching the duck, Katherine Rennie   121
Fumbling forward, Jessica Wachter   122

REFLECTIONS AND STORIES

Personal stories   124

Spiritual emergency:
Reflections of a mental health service user, David Norman   124
OCD: Faulty formulas, Thea Joshi   127
In the waiting, Thea Joshi   128
Anxiety, John Butterfield   129
My purple monster, Alex Clare-Young   130

Wounded healers   134

The rainbow man, Neil Paynter   134
Elizabeth, Neil Paynter   135
Maggie, Neil Paynter   135
George, Neil Paynter   136
Garry, Neil Paynter   138

The Bible   142

Blessed are the poor in spirit, Gill Dascombe   142
Ezekiel, Gill Dascombe   143
Consider the lilies of the field, Gill Dascombe   144
The Gerasene schizophrenic, Gill Dascombe   145
The woman who was bent double (Luke 13:10–13), Linda Hill   146
The aftermath of violence: Jephthah and his daughter, Rosemary Power   156
Contending with God (Genesis 32:22–32), Thom M Shuman   162
Waiting and hope, Thom M Shuman   164

Young people   166

A day in the life … Patrick: children and young people therapist,
    Patrick Bentley   166
Walking backwards … to savour the moment/Gary, Neil Squires and
    Jan Sutch Pickard   168
Waiting, Laura Gisbourne   171
Working therapeutically with young people during the pandemic,
    Susan Dale   173

A young man, Neil Paynter   175
The path, Katie Frost   176
David's story, Neil Paynter   176
A child at heart, Neil Paynter   179

Older people   182

Holy ground, Kathy Crawford   182
Nurse's notes, Neil Paynter   184
It smells like loneliness, Neil Paynter   189

Well-being   193

Burnout, Stephen G Wright   193
A Holy day, Bev Robertson   196
Well-being, John Butterfield   197
Loneliness makes you sick, Stephen G Wright   200
The goodness of nature, Rachel McCann   211
Cocoa the wonder dog, Thom M Shuman   214
Writing as therapeutic process, Susan Dale   216
Some things that make me feel better, Various   219

Community   220

Our mutual dependence, Iain Whyte   220
A psalm of hope, Christine Jones   221
Cyrenians: On supporting emotional and mental well-being during the pandemic and beyond, Ewan Aitken   223
A man has died, Alison Phipps   225
Musical hospitality, music-making and mental health, Jane Bentley   229
The Buddy Beat, Tom Chalmers   232
Pastoral conversation recollected, John Butterfield   233
The Asclepion of Pergamon, Gill Dascombe   234
Fellowship at the State Hospital, Philip Fox   235

About the authors   239

Sources and acknowledgements   245

Introduction

'One in four people will experience a mental health problem in their lifetime' is a statistic that is often quoted. Sometimes it's *'one in three'*, or *'one in two'*. While these are helpful stats, I think the reality is more like: *'Everyone in this overwhelming complicated difficult wonderful beautiful miracle of a world will experience a mental health problem at some point in their life.'* Why wouldn't we? Seems perfectly reasonable.

I have never known anyone who *hasn't* experienced a mental health problem at one time or another. I would *love* to meet the person who says they haven't. So, to me, this book is simply about being human. For example there are worship resources for services on mental health here, but I think a lot of the resources could, should be used in *any* worship service. And I hope some of it – the beautiful gutsy poems and powerful reflections – is used well beyond church. Much of it comes from the edge anyway. The book is also, I feel, a collective statement about mental health being, as the UN asserts, *'a human right'*.

I've not covered every aspect of mental health/well-being, of course, but the book does cover and touch on a lot. I hope it's helpful: creates conversations, more awareness, hope, community ...

If this book triggers any memories, thoughts, emotions, etc. you feel you want to talk to a mental health professional about, here are some possible resources:

British Association for Counselling and Psychotherapy: www.bacp.co.uk
Counselling & Psychotherapy in Scotland: www.cosca.org.uk
UK Council for Psychotherapy: www.psychotherapy.org.uk
(There will be similar organisations in some other countries.)

If you are needing help with your mental health, please reach out: to a friend, family, support worker, nurse, counsellor, the Samaritans (Tel: 116 123) ... This book itself is not that kind of resource. And I am not a mental health professional.

Thank you to everyone who contributed to *Redeeming Our Cracks*. Thank you for being so open, honest, generous, human ...

I'm sorry the book took a long time. Wild Goose is a small team, the book fell in the middle of covid, and then furloughs, and it just took a long time, the way some things in life and some books do. Thank you for your understanding and patience.

I have nothing very profound to say in this introduction about the subject of mental health and well-being, but if you read my little stories in the book you'll get some idea of where I've been and where I'm at.

Take care of yourself and each other.

Neil Paynter

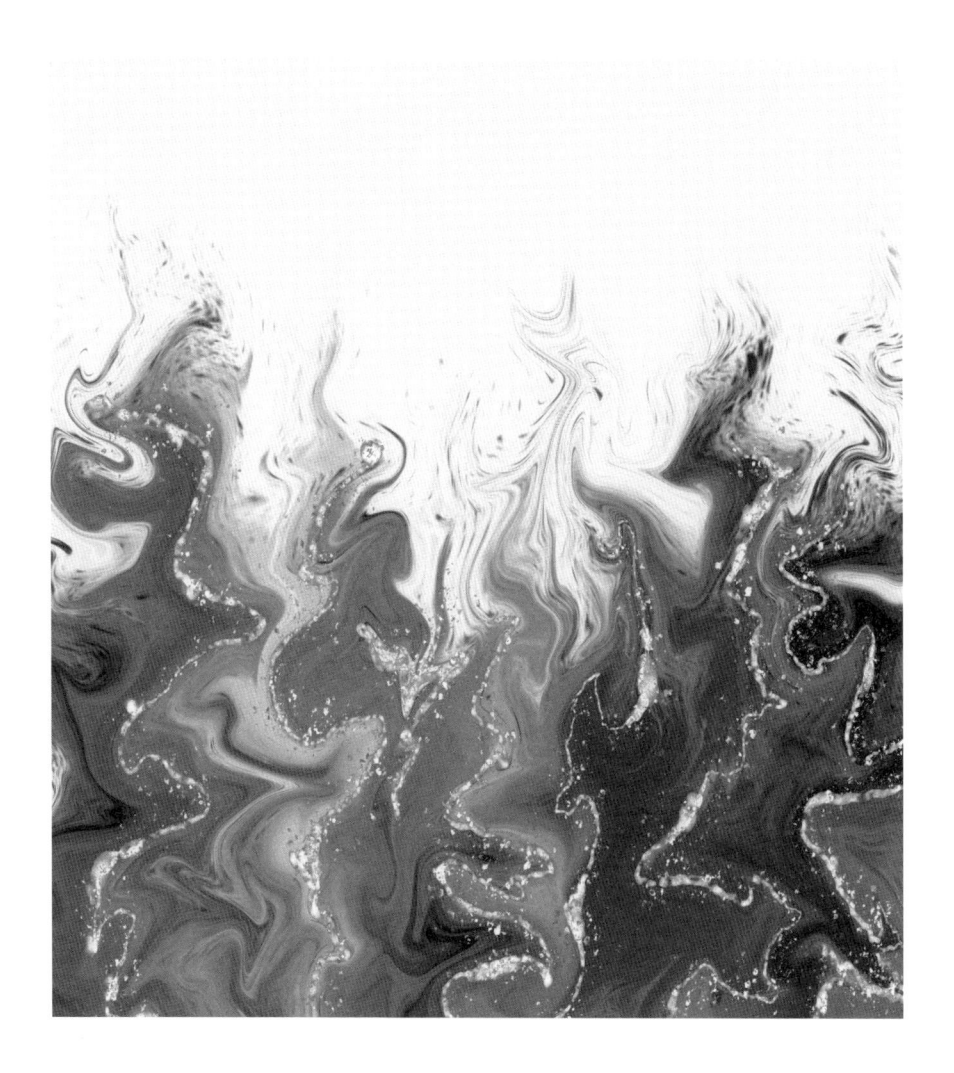

Prayers

Surprises and gifts

Cactus

When I am pressed into this corner,
paralysed with fear, Lord,
you come and sit with me and gently ask,
'What gift will you offer me?'
And all I can give you is a pot plant,
a cactus, to be precise,
very large,
with long, wicked spikes.
But then I find that you have anticipated my offering,
and have come crowned with thorns.
What love is this
that bedecks himself with my pain,
promising me the stars
away from this dark corner,
out there in the night sky?

Rev'd Sr Sandra Sears, CSBC

Surprising gifts

Life is tenacious, sometimes it has to be.
Parts of the old railway embankment
were set on fire;
it seemed as though
the plants stood no chance.
Some died.
But beneath the surface
new shoots stirred,
hanging on.
In time, they appeared,
pushing through
charred stems and ash,
as green and hopeful
as ever,

signs of spring,
unexpected,
a surprising gift.
Depression, chronic anxiety
burn up cherished hopes,
make a wasteland of plans
made in brighter moments.
But life is tenacious.
So, thankfully, are patience and love
in others who hold the Christ-light for us,
nurturing hope
that the future holds
surprising gifts.

Jesus, you were God's surprising gift to all of us, revealing the power of love and life to flower in the bleakest of circumstances. Help us not to give in or give up, and to find you in the friendship of others.

Jean Hudson

On mundane days

On mundane days it's easy to miss the thistledown
floating by on the breeze to settle and root elsewhere.
In commonplace spaces it's easy to overlook
the uncommon, small and rare things under stones.

In ordinary time it's easy to forget the extraordinary,
the surprises that creep up on us like sunrise.

As tiredness seeps into me
and weariness weighs me down,
it's easier to make my litany
from a limiting list of negatives
than a liberating whisper of possibilities.

In the still moment,
help me know
I can still be with you:

you are still here
and there are still surprises.

Janet Lees

Big Bang theory

Lord,
when my life blows apart
into a billion fragments,
remind me of that first moment,
when the wonder and spectacle
of all that surrounds me
began its journey into being,
and that every creative moment
begins with a big bang.
This too might just be the start
of something big,
something beautiful.

Rev'd Sr Sandra Sears, CSBC

Fragments

Lord,
you come,
walking among
the brittle fragments
of our broken lives,
gathering up every sharp shard,
to fashion
a new and beautiful
mosaic.
And all the while
your hands and feet
bleed for love of us.

Rev'd Sr Sandra Sears, CSBC

Still small voice

God of the still small voice,
you speak to us
when we least expect it;

we hear your voice
in moments of
chaos, clutter and uncertainty.

Jesus, calmer of the storms,
your very presence comforts us;

we are upheld
by your quiet authority.

Spirit, Counsellor,
carrier of our pain and celebrations,
we gather under your cloak of soft down
and sharp flight-feathers;

we feel the flutterings
of the longings to be born.

Elizabeth Baxter

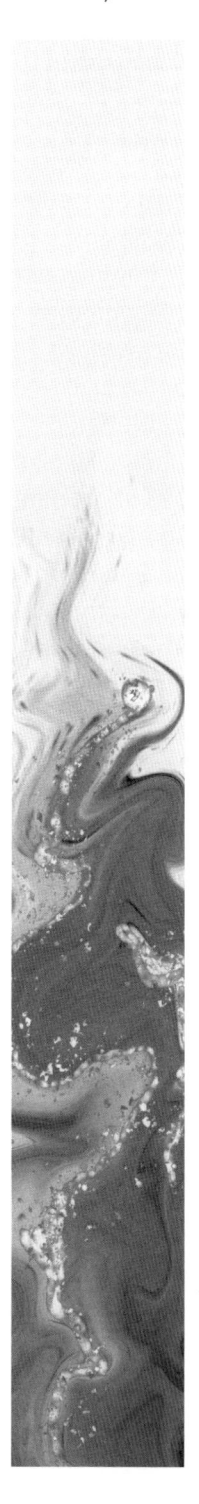

Community

Swallows

Getting ready
for an epic journey.
For us it would be
the journey of a lifetime;
for swallows
an annual event.
But it is not
undertaken lightly –
lots of preening,
short, exploratory flights,
and, most importantly,
gathering together.
The epic flight
is made in a flock,
together.
We like to think
we are
self-sufficient.
But alone can soon become
lonely,
tedious,
limiting.
Better together –
stimulating,
creative,
encouraging,
healing.

God, you bind the whole world to yourself. Teach us to be unafraid of the cost of loving and being loved. Save us from isolation of our own or others' making.

Jean Hudson

A lineup for the exhausted

Pugh, Pugh, Barney McGrew, Cuthbert, Dibble, Grubb:
all lined up, ready for anything.
After several weeks of firefighting,
there's nothing else coming out.
I'm like Dibble:
I can stand next in the line,
hold out my hose in hope,
but just like Dibble,
I don't have a dribble.

God of grace,
of mercy and compassion,
revive us drop by drop.

(Pugh and the others were a famous set of firefighters in a children's TV programme.)

Janet Lees

A prayer for real church

We give thanks to you, gracious Lord,
that our relationship with you is not superficial or shallow.
You know us like no one else;
we try hard to hide much from others
but nothing is hidden from you,
so we might as well be open and honest with you.
You know all our brokenness;
you are aware of our frailty and vulnerability.
Yet still in your kindness and love
you invite us into your presence
and welcome us into your family.

We pray that our church
will be characterised by this real and authentic love.

Let us accept one another with our imperfections
and be aware that we have struggled and failed.
Let us not be blind to our weaknesses and our battles
but face them together.

May our church show patience and understanding,
tolerate the questions we ask
and go on welcoming and accepting.

May this community of God's children
be a safe place where we know we belong,
know that we are loved
and in that love find a deep, inner healing.

In receiving and giving kindness,
may this church transform lives.
May we be a new community,
characterised by a love that forgives,
liberates
and hopes beyond hope.
Amen

Simon Taylor

Alyas' prayer

From Iona Community member Susan Dale:

I met Alyas when I stayed on Iona for a week as 'Member in Residence', supporting the guests and staff. We started to talk over a cup of tea in the refectory one evening after a service. Later, she e-mailed me a copy of a prayer which she had left in the south aisle of the Abbey Church. Since then we have been in regular correspondence. Alyas wanted me to include her prayer here, as she feels that staying on Iona, and writing this, was a turning point in her life:

Why, God, have you put me, a Christian,
into the body of an Asian transgender woman?
I call myself Alyas – 'brave one',
but I wish that I did not have to be, or that I was more so.

Why do other Christians exclude, deride and humiliate me?
Which part of the Gospel message says:
I have to be 'cured' rather than loved?
Why do they pray over me, rather than with me?

Where are you, Lord, when I need you?
Alienated now from my family, my birth sex and religion.
Where do I find help?
I found hope for a while on Iona.
For a week, the sea, the white sand,
space to be me.
The love of people around me
allowed a glimpse of what it may mean to be myself
and part of God's family,
accepted for who I am.

Thank you, God, for this place, these people.
Give me the courage to make changes in my life.

Alyas, while a guest at the MacLeod Centre, 2014

At times like this

My God,
at times you're hard to believe in,
when hell comes closest
and hope seems to trickle into the ground.

At times like this,
may the smallest spark of love,
seen in the outstretched hand,
keep us alive to your presence in us all,
and may that give us the will to believe.

Janet Lees

Dove of Peace

This prayer was originally written for folk at the Palace Gate Centre, a community centre run by South Street Baptist Church in Exeter. The Centre is used by people experiencing mental health difficulties, emotional problems or recovering from addiction.

Dove of Peace,
life-giving Spirit of God,
touch the lives of each who come into this place,
that all may find refuge under your wings of love.
In sharing our hurt
may we journey towards healing;

in sharing our vulnerability
may we find new strength;

in sharing ourselves
may we support one another;

in letting go of our burdens,
may we be able to begin again.

Glide through all offered within these walls,
that here we may find a deeper well-being in our lives
and the still calm of your peace,
through Jesus our Friend and Saviour.
Amen

Simon Taylor

Calling disciples

We are unable to speak up:
You sit with us in silence.

We think we are alone:
You affirm us as friends.

We seem buried in hopelessness:
You wait beside us, ready to rise.

We feel excluded:
You include us.

Our lives are in turmoil:
You say 'Go in peace.'

Janet Lees

Breath prayer

Breathe in the breath of God.
Breathe out your cares and concerns …

Breathe in the love of God.
Breathe out your doubts and despair …

Breathe in the life of God.
Breathe out your fears and frustrations …

**We sit quietly before the One
who gives life and love to all creation.**

**We sit in awe of the One
who formed us in our mother's womb.**

**We sit at peace, surrounded by the One
who fills every fibre of our being …**

Breathe in the breath of God.
Breathe out your tensions and turmoil …

Breathe in the peace of God.
Breathe out your haste and hurry …

Breathe in the delights of God.
Breathe out your pain …

In the forgiveness of God,
we live and move and have our being.

Through the healing touch of Christ,
we find ourselves beloved.
In solidarity with all who seek human flourishing,
we leave behind our faithlessness and our fearfulness,
working humbly together
towards health and healing in our community,
our churches
and the world around us.

Elizabeth Baxter

Rising Christa

I celebrate your rising,
beloved Christa.
You have not abandoned me.

Speak to me,
call me by my name;
allow me to touch
and heal your wounds,
to feel your breath
come into me
and I will find my voice.
I will sing your song of freedom
and eternal presence.
You befriend us
into community,
gathering abandoned chaos,
transforming pain
into songs of angels,
opening the way
of friendship.

Elizabeth Baxter

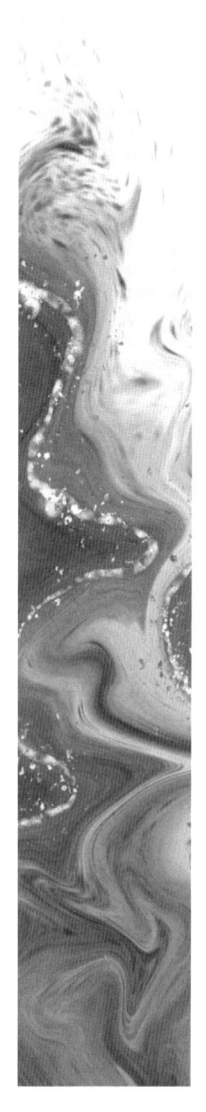

Prayers of concern

Prayer for all with invisible illnesses

We pray for all with invisible illnesses.
A broken leg we can see,
a fever we can feel,
but when the illness is deep inside,
inside the body or the mind,
it is invisible to us all.
We see only symptoms:
uncharacteristic behaviours,
lack of energy,
looking drawn or tired,
being irritable or rude.

Lord, we pray for those suffering from invisible illnesses.
May we not judge others based on what we see.

Bring healing, hope, peace and love,
that all may be surrounded by positives
and not suffer from an invisible illness alone.
Amen

John Butterfield

God of healing and wholeness (based on Psalm 116:5)

You could adapt this to the specific needs of your congregation/community.

**The Lord is gracious and righteous.
Our God is full of compassion.**

Father God, it's because we realise how much you care
and want the best for each of us
that we have the confidence to pray for those in need of your healing.
We know that you are able to fathom our deepest thoughts and emotions,
even when we ourselves cannot understand them,
or find the words to express how we feel.

The Lord is gracious and righteous.
Our God is full of compassion.

We pray for all who have suffered any kind of loss in their lives
and who are struggling to make sense of what has happened.
We ask that, in their grief and confusion,
you give them a continual awareness of your presence
and the strength they need to face the future with hope.

The Lord is gracious and righteous.
Our God is full of compassion.

We remember people suffering from post-traumatic stress disorder,
whose sleep is regularly disrupted by flashbacks of distressing things
they have seen or situations they have experienced.
May they find understanding, help and support
to confront their nightmares
and discover once more
a sense of peace.

The Lord is gracious and righteous.
Our God is full of compassion.

We pray for all those who have been the victims of abuse or bullying
and are suffering mental, emotional or physical scars as a result.
We ask that you would begin to heal their brokenness
and restore their self-esteem.
Give them inner strength and the ability
to recognise people whom they can genuinely trust.

The Lord is gracious and righteous.
Our God is full of compassion.

We remember everybody who is anxious or afraid
of what the future may bring.
Especially we think of those who are undergoing medical treatment,
waiting for test results,
or caring for someone with a terminal illness …

The Lord is gracious and righteous.
Our God is full of compassion.

We pray for people whose lives are ruled by alcohol,
drug or substance abuse;
for those who treat it as a way of deadening their depression and pain,
easing their loneliness, or avoiding the challenges of daily life;
for those who become aggressive
when they are unable to feed their addiction.
While we admit we sometimes feel these situations are hopeless,
we know you can still see the potential in people and,
like a loving father,
you wait longingly for your prodigal children to come home.

The Lord is gracious and righteous.
Our God is full of compassion.

God of healing and wholeness,
God, the source of hope and love,
we commit all those we know who suffer mentally and emotionally,
for whatever reason,
to your loving care.
Amen

Kathy Crawford

A prayer for those who offer pastoral care

Understanding God,
I feel at my most useless
when alongside those who are in deep depression
or tipping over the edge into harmful thoughts and acts.
It's not them, it's me.
I know they would not choose to be where they are.

Sitting there with one lost in unending despair,
tears falling down a silent face,
I do not know the words that will bring them through.

Alongside one who speaks eagerly and with passion,
yet with phrases that make no sense,
I do not know how to bring them home.

Waiting in Accident and Emergency,
as doctors and nurses assess the damage done,
I cannot find a way to make them feel better about themselves.

Simplistic notions of healing
that do not know the complexity of their pain
will not make them well.

My naive prayers seem so inadequate
as I struggle to bring their situation to God
and God's peace to their mind.

All I can do is be there,
sometimes alongside,
often at the end of the phone.

All I can do is be there,
to hold on to a hand,
to reassure that they are valued,
tell them that they are loved
and to patiently and persistently
show they matter.

All I can do is to go on being there,
and hope and pray
that this will be enough.

Lord, I trust that you will be there,
with me and for them,
and this will be enough.

Simon Taylor

God of community

God of community
present with us
in our brokenness;

you embrace us here,
gathering our fragmented lives,
restoring us with new hope.

Teach us to live gently with our sorrows,
to find solidarity with others,
and our own resources for healing.

God of compassion,
we pray for all people
who live today with fear, hunger,
sickness and loss.

In your tenderness enfold them.
In your justice bring them hope.
In your mercy forgive us
for our part in the injustices of the world.
Amen

Elizabeth Baxter

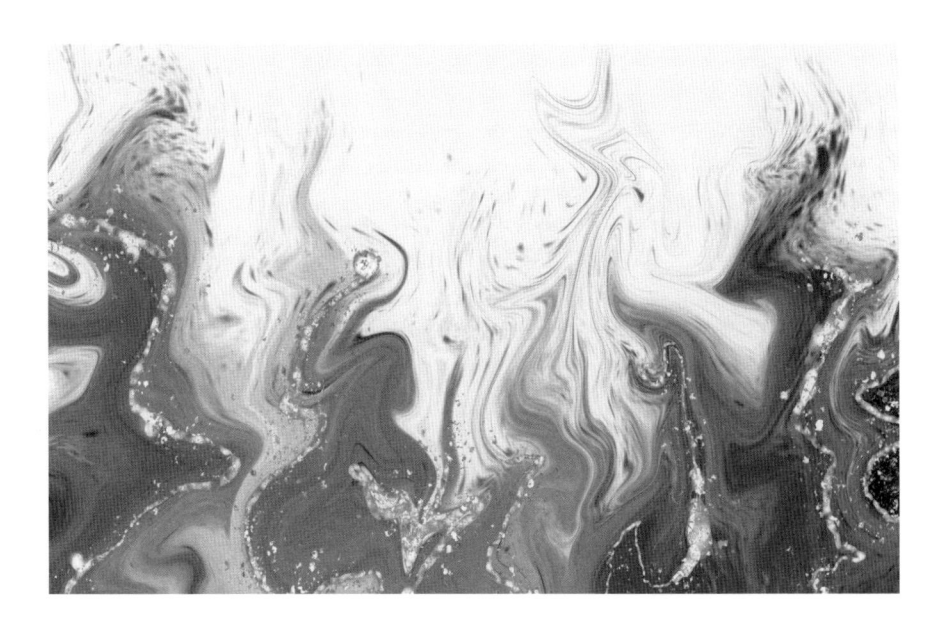

Prayer for ourselves

Gentle God,
close to me,
hold me in your love;

bring strength
when I feel weak;

bring courage
when I feel despair;

bring peace
when I feel afraid.

Jesus, healer,
be my companion through my pain;
hold my hand through suffering;

walk beside me
to steady me;

before me
to guide me;

behind me
lest I fall.

Compassionate Spirit,
alert me to your call;

inspire me to share

your passion,
your wisdom,
your justice,
to bring healing to the world.

Elizabeth Baxter

Darkness and light

The evening draws on

As we gather together
while the evening draws on
and the night begins to fall,
we gather with us those
who are afraid of the night-time,
and those who are waking to a new dawn.

Elizabeth Baxter

The night draws in

Strong and lovely one,
gather up our weariness;
free up our heaviness.

As the night draws in
the Spirit wafts her way through the shadows,
integrating light and darkness;
beaming her presence;
opening up our possibilities
for tomorrow.

Elizabeth Baxter

Dying darkness

If I can die into the darkness –
the deep night of fear,
the black hole that threatens
to suck the life out of me –
if I can die into the darkness
I find myself in a womb,
surrounded by love,

soothed by the heartbeat of God
resonating through my very being,
nurtured and fed,
shaped and formed,
until I am strong enough
to be born once more into new life,
new light.

Rev'd Sr Sandra Sears, CSBC

Calling One (A psalm)

Calling One, has your love been exhausted?
Mine has in so many ways and places.
I only seem to have a little left
and in itself that is painful to me,
when I remember all the love-filled times and places
and compare them with this pitiful situation.

I am sad, and have been for some time:
sad enough to be sick, and sick of sadness,
but unable to leave sadness behind.
I have left the church of my youth behind me:
I opened the doors and stepped outside.
Although I was called 'a breath of fresh air'
I heard the door bang shut behind me.

I am exhausted from lamenting all of this:
my love has poured out onto hard ground,
soaked into the parched cracks and is gone.
It is not just my eyes that weep,
but every part of me feels heavy;
my guts twist and turn, my back aches from the load.
How I wish I could put down this sorrow and leave this pain behind.

As I go out each morning, ready for each new encounter,
I know I am fortunate to meet those who yearn to know you:
a child comes running towards me,
a youth begins a conversation

and each time my heart takes a joyful jump.
When we sing together or remember the stories,
then my heart glows warm again.

Calling One,
your love has not been exhausted;
I rejoice that it is new every morning.

Janet Lees

Prayer from a prayer-writing workshop at Dove Café

Dove Café is a community café run by South Street Baptist Church in central Exeter, with support from the Devon NHS Partnership. It is well-used by people who are coping with long-term mental health issues.

You come to me

Lord, You come to me
when I am in a dark place –
and You make it Light.

Lord, You come to me
when all is Light
and You make that place Warm.

Lord, You come to me
when all is Light and Warm
and You bring Peace.

Lord, may I always worship
and serve You
and bring Your Light
and Warmth and Peace
to those I meet.

Susan Palmer

Healing prayer

Healing God,
Source of peace and calm,
Source of life in all its fullness and fountain of health:
> re-balance what has become muddled
> re-align what is not where it should be
> re-shape what has morphed into disorder.

Holy Spirit,
Spirit of fire and water and power,
Spirit of healing:
Send your blazing light
> to make right all that is wrong in us
> heal all that is broken
> and calm all that is troubled.

In the name of the Blessed Trinity,
God the Father, God the Son and God the Holy Spirit.
Amen

John Butterfield

Scars

They tell me
that scars fade
over time
but they don't.

They tell me
that hurt belongs
to the past
but it doesn't.

They tell me
that I should forget
but I can't.

They tell me
to soldier on
but I'm too exhausted.

They tell me
there's a light
at the end of the tunnel
but this tunnel
is too long.

They tell me
to think positively
but I can't see
through this darkness.

They tell me
that I'm just
a hopeless case.
Ah! Now I think
they're right
but every time I do that
my scars itch and prick
and won't leave me alone
even though
they should have faded
long ago.

Estranged from them
(those who tell me)
in my isolation
I crave …
long for …
wonder
if I will ever know …
the company of one
who understands,
who won't just tell me stuff.

One who hurts
like me.
One who wears,
shares,
bears
my scars.

Rev'd Sr Sandra Sears, CSBC

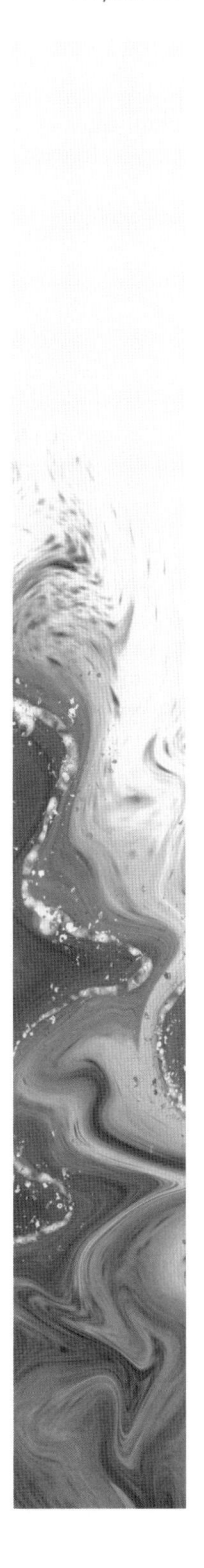

Still praying

Most days,
it's just about all I can do.

Janet Lees

An Easter prayer

Come, liberating Christ,
rise to meet us!
Banish the darkness of our fears.
Release us from our tombs of powerlessness
into empowered living
in the movement
of your liberating Spirit.

God of all life and empowerment,
who through the resurrection of Jesus
opened a new way
out of the tombs of oppression
into a garden of beauty,
grant that we may no longer cling
to our grave clothes;
the familiar comfort that holds us back;
but call us out
and empower us
to be alive to one another
so we may bear witness to the movement of the Spirit
and the flourishing of the whole world.
Amen

Elizabeth Baxter

Like the catkins

A beautiful
blue breezy day
ideal for seeing
catkins.
Catkins make me smile.
They are so iconic:
a sign of spring
and returning life.
They actually
appear in December,
and can be seen
with icicles attached,
against a backdrop
of deep snow.
But on a day like this
they come into their own,
flying high on the breeze.
Even though my current
plodding pace is at odds
with such flying freedom
I begin to hope
that one day
it will be different,
that tiny spurts of
creative energy
that often come to
nothing
will gain
momentum
and I will
fly high
like the catkins.

Infinite God of skies and breezes and freedom, help us, even when we feel burdened and limited, to hope that one day we will reach for the stars, become the people we dream of being.

Jean Hudson

Dance of life

We name ourselves
in the dance of life.
As a butterfly flutters from hidden space,
so we are freed from hiding.

As flowers stand tall,
each with dignity,
together in solidarity,
so they call us to do the same.

We can come out
to be ourselves,
to play with others,
to enter into our becoming,
to dance new steps,
feeling grass on bare feet
and softness of skin.

Playful God,
hues of colour
evoke our senses,
branches wave to us
calling us to dance.

Release us from our fears,
renew our energies
and restore our joy.

Elizabeth Baxter

Still calling

In joy and sorrow,
in gain and loss,
in despair and hope,
in death and life,
the Constant One
calls me still.

Janet Lees

Prayer of re-turn

Restore me to my soul,
to the gentle breath of being,
unravel my entangled mind
from knots of obligation.
Let me open this tight fist of self
like a lotus sensing the sun.

Re-member this dismemberment
of fractured, forgotten life
in the light of your seeing.
Where my focus of meaning is
more than sound-bite insanity
and the pushing and pulling
of blind unknowing.

Bring me again to the sacred soil of my soul
deep in the waters of Being,
where the eye can see and the heart can sense
the vastness of Love's simplicity.

Bev Robertson

Journeying prayer

God of vision,
present with us in our journeying,
teach us to integrate
the light and shadow of our lives,
to feel more at home within ourselves.

Elizabeth Baxter

Phos Hilaron (O gracious Light!)

O gracious Light!
Pure brightness of the ever-living Father in heaven,
kindling my dollar-store candle
and firing up the fluorescent fixtures,
you turn my evensong into the Inner Sanctum,
my fingers to your altars.

Now as we come to the setting of the sun
(mass incarceration and violent deportation
and nuclear proliferation and clinical depression
and generalised anxiety and the decline of the
institutional church and the death of Christendom
and the rise of technological addiction and the dawn
of climate change and the extinction of civilisation
and my debt to income ratio and my check engine
light and elevated body mass index and stripes of greying
hair and the dearth of eligible bachelors with acceptable
political leanings and I am almost out of eggs).

Now. My eyes behold the vesper light –
flame twirling, flame spinning, upright and at attention
in anticipation I am going to say something,
yet (don't touch!) the impenetrable pinprick
between this world and the next.

You who rejoice at my dark and feeble presence,
you who are ever-living, ever-singing,
you who still my chatter
with silence –

you who made, who are the Light –

you're worthy at all times to be praised by happy voices.

Jessica Wachter

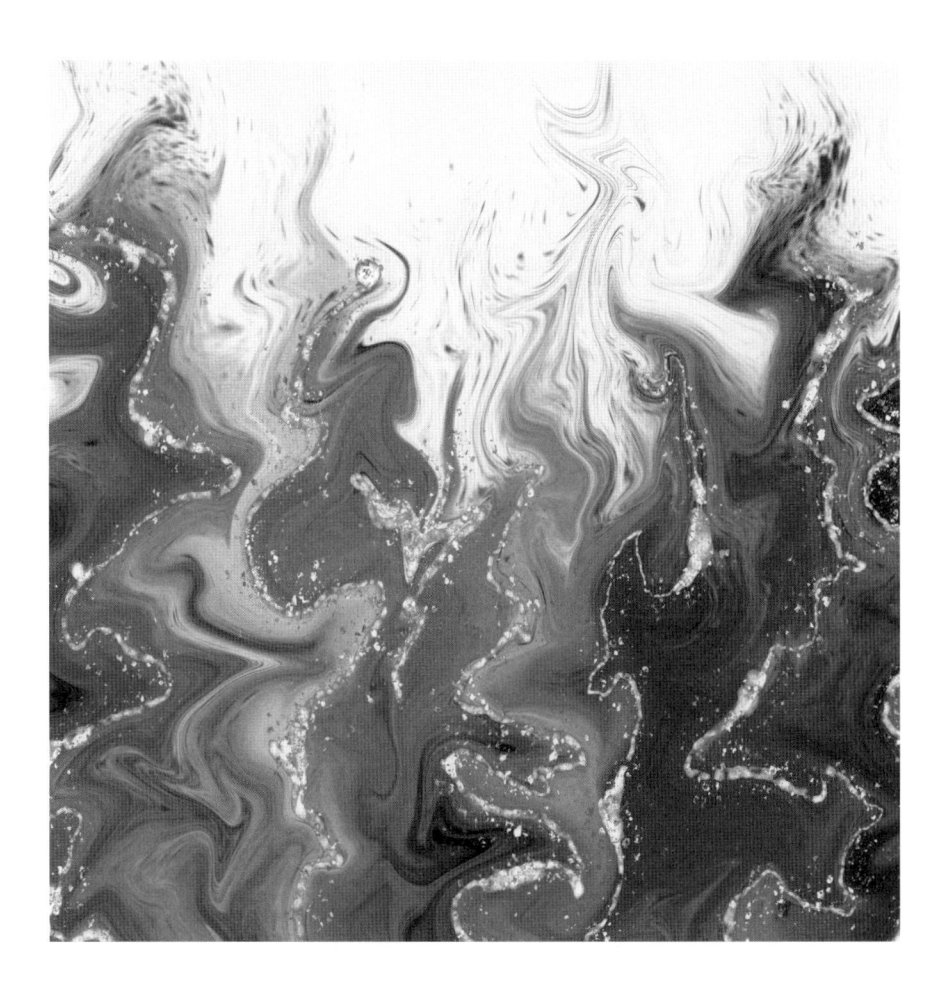

Prayers of thanksgiving and praise

Every day

Dear Lord Jesus,
I thank you because
I know that no burden of mine
is too big
or too small
for you to help me carry.
You lead and guide and strengthen me
through every experience
and the joy of walking with you
surpasses every trouble.
My soul rejoices in Jesus, my Saviour,
every day.

Susan Palmer, at Dove Café

In emotional turmoil

Dear God,
my mind's in a whirl; my head's spinning;
I'm not sure if my feet are on the ground
or if I'm existing on a different plane;
but you are my stable ground wherever I am,
ground that will shift with me
so that I will not disappear down a deep chasm.
I need you; I am so thankful that you are real
and not a figment of my imagination –
though I know I don't always have even this trust.
When things are out of my hands, hold on to me;
keep me and my loved ones, whom I name now, safe …

May we all be happy,
and as well as it's possible

for each of us to be.
Thank you.
Amen

Pamela Turner

Beginning to emerge from bereavement

Thank you, God, for this new day.
Thank you, God, that I can pray.
Thank you for the sun's arising.
Thank you that I'm more than surviving.

Katy Owen

Thank you for old friends

God, thank you for the old friends I turn to
when I am feeling alone and crazy:

Thank you for Henri Nouwen
for Vincent Van Gogh
for Sylvia Plath
for Henry David Thoreau
for William Blake
for Tennessee Williams
for Allen Ginsberg …

God, thank you for the old friends I turn to
when I am feeling alone and crazy.

Old friends who restore my sanity and hope.
Old friends who give me the inspiration and passion
to live and love again.

Neil Paynter

A psalm of thanksgiving

God, I feel I could wear the day
I feel I could wear the day today
like a scarf
(But not because it's cold
'cause it's not)
I feel I could wear the day and
the wind would wrap it around and around me
I feel I could wear the day
I feel I could wear the day today
Like a scarf
and dance it
Yellow with a fringe or two of blue …

Neil Paynter

Examine me

I thank you, Creator, for dappled sunlight and drawn curtains.
I thank you, Jesus, for remembered encounters and forgotten ones.
I thank you, Spirit, for energy for life and for when it runs out.
Show me now the way I should go.

Christ in joy
Christ in pain
Christ in turmoil
Christ in love
Christ in anger
Christ in harmony
Christ in anxiety
Christ in freedom
Christ in captivity
Christ in company
Christ in isolation
Christ in all

Like a ray of light through a magnifying glass, focus me, God:
may I be attentive and listening.
And as for tomorrow, as I feel my way,
may I rise again.

Janet Lees

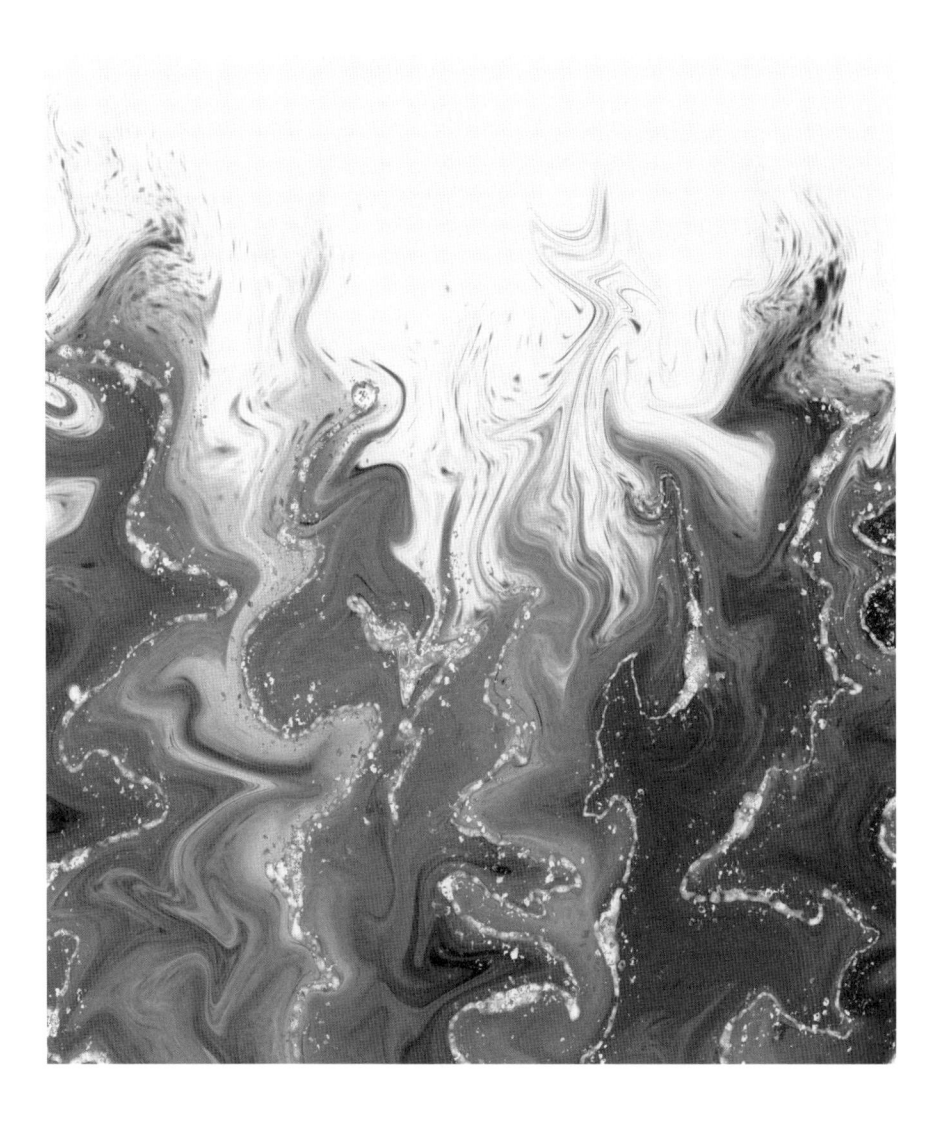

Prayers for protection, safety, comfort and rest

Prayer for protection

Draw a circle around yourself, from your heart, up and over your head and back to your heart. Imagine this as a welcoming hug, protecting and enfolding. Do this for the first three stanzas of the prayer.

In the second half of the prayer, imagine, in your mind's eye, God's love, peace, protection encircling the person you name.

God, circle me around with love:
holding, helping, healing.

Circle me around with peace:
caressing, caring, comforting.

Circle me around with protection:
guarding, guiding, giving …
hope.

God, circle *(name)* around with love:
holding, helping, healing.

Circle *(name)* around with peace:
caressing, caring, comforting.

Circle *(name)* around with protection:
guarding, guiding, giving …
hope.

Elizabeth Baxter

A safe place

Lord,
help me to find
a safe place
where I can rest;
a place where I feel secure
and can find a moment of peace
away from the demands on me,
the problems I don't know how to solve,
and the people I sometimes just can't cope with.

It might be
a bench in the park,
green space amongst the urban roar;
a tree by a river
where the water sings and the leaves whisper;
a corner in a favourite café,
with tea and toast to comfort and warm;
or hiding under the duvet,
that soothing cotton barrier
protecting from the world outside.

Meet me there;
hold me there in your love for me.
Let anxiety slip away,
and in stillness
may I know a moment
that is simply quiet …

Then give me the strength
to go back to my day,
reassured that the God
who meets me in my safe place,
walks with me in the places
that are loud and stressful.

Simon Taylor

We come, Holy One

From fear,
        from misery,
                from worry,
we come, Holy One.

From despair,
        from remorse,
                from regret,
from the valley of the shadow, in which we live, and move,
and have our being,
we come.

From exhaustion,
        from torment,
                from distress,
we come, Creator of all.

Dwarfed by mountains impossible to see past or climb over,
        without rest or sleep, with anxiety and trepidation,
                in mental anguish, physical pain,
we come.

Alone and lonely, running on empty,
        clothed in sackcloth, dripping ashes,
                living greyscale lives in a kaleidoscope world,
we come, Sacred Presence.

From brokenness,
        from infirmity,
                from sorrow,
        our words turning to dust in our throats
before we can utter them,
we come, casting ourselves on your mercy.

Deliver us, Holy One, whose eye is on even the sparrow,
        from night terrors and day arrows.

Breathe life into our dry-bones existence,
>> bind up our wounds of body and mind and spirit,
>>>> ease the pain unleashed on us from outside,
and from within.

Pour your healing balm upon our bruised and broken hearts.
>> Speak peace to our frayed tempers, our frazzled nerves.

Surprise us with unexpected graces in the wilderness of our days:
>> bread and wine, milk and honey.
>>>> Slake our thirst with life-giving water of your Spirit.

Hear our prayer, O Lord, our Rock, our Refuge, our Strong Tower,
our Safe Space.

Silence

Words of assurance:

In unfailing love and endless mercy, the Sacred meets us here.
The One who knows all hearts sees and acknowledges every scattered and anxious thought,
>> each moment of despair, every tear shed and sorrow mourned,
>>>> and offers grace and peace, courage and strength, life
and hope.

You, who are both Breath of Heaven and dust of the earth,
>> fearfully and wonderfully made,
>>>> are Beloved of God, welcomed and heard.

Rest in the presence of the Holy,
knowing you are loved and accepted just as you are.

Kathy Swaar

God's cushions

God's grace and mercy
are cushions on which I rest.
Right now,
I can do nothing else.

Janet Lees

Angel of the North

The Angel of the North is a sculpture by Antony Gormley, in Gateshead, Tyne and Wear, England.

Why are angels so flimsy and feminine
always?
I need strong steel.
I need your giant frame,
your wonderfully wide wings
right for embracing on earth
rather than taking flight into heaven.

Stand tall for me, God,
as I brace for storms;
steel me for my next step in life.
Embrace me now
with your grounded heavenly love.
Please.
Amen

Pamela Turner

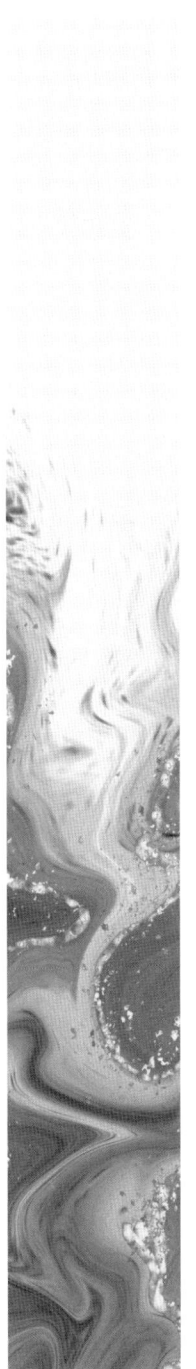

The promise

Bare branches
where, in spring,
buds gave birth
to leaves;
where, in this abundant autumn,
bright red berries
provided food for birds,
pretty to look at.
Now all life is
apparently
spent.
We can feel like that
when life changes …
relationships interrupted
with partner, children,
colleagues, friends,
sometimes abruptly
ending.
Loss of purpose, drive,
identity, reason for living.
But closer inspection of the tree
reveals buds
dormant for now
but nurturing new life
for another spring.
Energy,
love,
life
might lie dormant
while we adjust
to unwelcome
change.
But they hold
the promise
of a new flowering,

too powerful,
too precious
to waste.

Jesus, you welcome the weary and nurture the downhearted. Help us to rest in order to be set free to live again.

Jean Hudson

Soothe me, Lord

Soothe me, Lord,
with your calming voice and gentle presence.

Still me, Lord,
so my heartbeat is steadied
by being at one with yours.
Guide me forward into a place
where I can hold my head high,
eyes no longer downcast.
Hold me in your loving gaze when I waiver.
Stand and watch me
as I step forward in freedom.

Ann Jepson

The answer

There is a whispered answer I hear when I'm depressed,
when anxious thoughts engulf me and I feel I'm so hard-pressed.

Or if I'm hypermanic, with psychotic symptoms too,
the answer comes through others' care, the healing things they do.

For in Him we have the answer, who is there whate'er betide;
he brightens up our darkness, as He shines His Light inside. *(Jn 1)*

He clothes us in His armour, lets His strength our weakness hide; *(Eph 6)*
and the fiery darts aimed at us He will scatter far and wide.

In the storms that so assail us He is always at our side;
we will find our hearts can trust Him, and in peace we can abide. *(Mk 4)*

For the threatening dark around us can no more be felt or eyed,
and the rising fears within us will recede as ebbs the tide.

David Norman

Holy Spirit

Enabler
Protector
Counsellor
Prompter
Healer
Teacher

Multiple aspects
Myriad descriptions
Personal experiences
Complex situations

Giver of life
Light in the dark
Guide to the lost
Warmth in the cold
Breath to the stressed
At work in the world

Emma Major

Blessings

A blessing for those who are depressed

God be with all those who are depressed.
Bless them with the support
and understanding
of friends and family,
and be close to those without family or friends.
Protect them, sheltering God,
and help them make their home in you.

Neil Paynter

Blessing for a carer

May God give you the strength to get through today without becoming totally exhausted.

May you have the wisdom and ability to deal calmly with any crises.

May you somehow find the patience to answer, yet again, the same question you were asked five minutes ago, and five minutes before that, and five minutes before that …

May you have a good sense of humour to enable you to laugh quietly to yourself about situations that in some ways are also poignantly sad.

May you continue to show a deep, genuine love that overrides all sense of duty and irritating behaviour.

May you not bottle up your emotions or believe it's a sign of weakness to express frustration – especially when you are tired.

May you never feel guilty that your humanity means that all you can offer anyone is your best.

May happy memories of the life you've shared still bring smiles to your face, and gently outweigh the pain when the one with whom you've shared so much sometimes forgets your name.

May you find the support you need from people who understand what you're going through: the ones who can always find time to put the kettle on; the friends who are never embarrassed when life gets too much and you suddenly burst into tears.

And, in the busyness of caring, may you always remember that you have a Heavenly Father who values the person you are and will lovingly care for you.

Kathy Crawford

A blessing for those who have no one left to talk to

Listening God, bless all those
who have no one left to talk to,
who are afraid
friends will reject them,
families will disown them
and lovers will leave.

Bless them with the confidence, loving God,
that no matter what they confess
you love and accept them,
understand their shadow and their light,
will never leave them feeling ashamed, poor, alone.

Neil Paynter

Bless us

When we are happy,
when we feel your presence,
when the sun shines on us,
bless us.

When we are sad,
when we cannot find you,
when the rain keeps on falling,
bless us.

Bless us,
with tears and laughter,
with courage and curiosity,
with hope and healing.

Bless us with love.

Ruth Burgess

Give me a smile

Give me a smile, God.

Look me in the eye
and give me your blessing.

Bless me in mind and in body.

Look on me with love.

Ruth Burgess

When

Bless us when we're cheerful.
Bless us when we're upset.
Bless us with healing and hope.

Bless us when we're relaxed.
Bless us when we're anxious.
Bless us with healing and trust.

Bless us when we're calm.
Bless us when we're angry.
Bless us with healing and peace.

Bless us when we're joyful.
Bless us when we're weary.
Bless us with healing and strength.

Bless us when we lie awake.
Bless us when we're sleeping.
Bless us with wonder, healing and love.

Ruth Burgess

Along the roads and byways

Bless us in our good days.
Bless us in our bad days.

Bless us with friends and family.
Bless us with strangers.
Bless us with trees and dandelions.
Bless us with city streets and cafés.
Bless us with storytellers and buskers.
Bless us with weeping and with joy.

Bless us, God, with healing and adventure
along the roads and byways
of our journey home.

Ruth Burgess

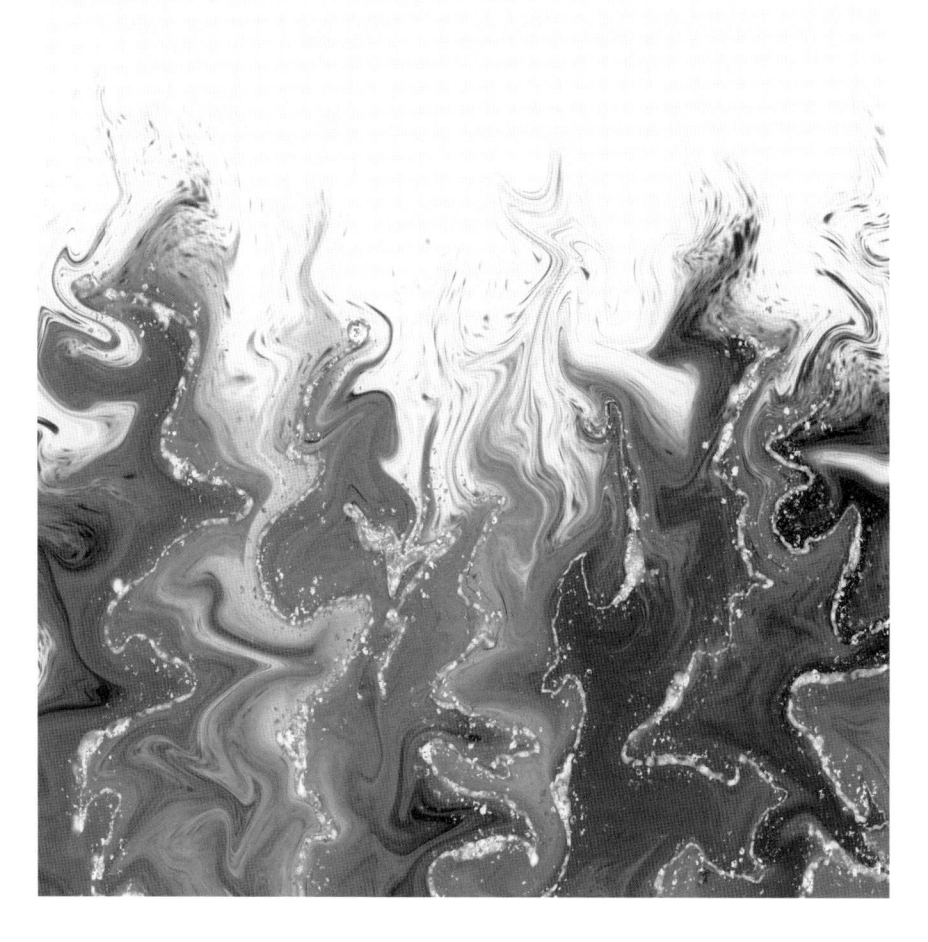

Redeeming our cracks

A liturgy on changing perspectives on mental ill health

For this liturgy you will need: plain sheets of paper, coloured pens, crayons, poster paints, magazine images of pottery (which can be torn to create 'cracks' or 'brokenness'), and strips of paper and pens. These can be handed out, placed centrally, etc. You will also need a central table with a large candle on it.

Introduction:

'… 1 in 4 people will experience a mental health problem each year.'
Statistic from MIND, a mental health charity (www.mind.org.uk)

Despite how common mental health problems are, stigmatising behaviour and language towards those experiencing mental ill health is still very prevalent.

We reject what we fear.

But this rejection overlooks and ignores the rich source of understanding, compassion and wisdom we could draw on, if only we would open up to what those who have travelled the hard roads before us can teach us.

'He's cracked.' 'She's cracking up.' 'They're all cracked.' 'The cracks are showing' … This imagery is fairly 'innocuous' – at least in comparison to much of the language often hurled at people because of their mental ill health in places like on social media.

But let's take some time in this service to reflect on whether we can discover any positive aspects in the image of cracks.

Prayer for insight:

God of our daily lives,
we know that we are created in your image –
fearfully and wonderfully made,
every individual included in your generous outpouring of
grace and mercy.

We confess that we have sometimes excluded our sisters and brothers
from the full bounty of your table and
the freedom of your loving community,
and, in silence, we ask your forgiveness …

Help us, as we reflect on those times in our lives
when our thoughts, language and actions
have fallen short of what you require of us:

'to do justice,
and to love kindness,
and to walk humbly with you'. *(Micah 6:8)*

Silence, during which gentle music could be played as people reflect.

Creative meditation:

First, some wisdom from the East:

'*Kintsugi* (or *Kintsukuroi*, which means "golden repair") is the centuries-old Japanese art of fixing broken pottery with a special lacquer dusted with powdered gold, silver or platinum. Beautiful seams of gold glint in the cracks of ceramic ware, giving a unique appearance to the piece.

This repair method celebrates each artefact's unique history by emphasising its fractures and breaks, instead of hiding or disguising them. *Kintsugi* often makes the repaired piece even more beautiful than the original, revitalising it with new life …

Since its conception, *Kintsugi* has been heavily influenced by prevalent philosophical ideas. Namely, the practice is related to the Japanese philosophy of *wabi-sabi*, which calls for seeing beauty in the flawed or imperfect. The repair method was also born from the Japanese feeling of *mottainai*, which expresses regret when something is wasted, as well as *mushin*, the acceptance of change.'[1]

Look at some examples of Kintsugi (or Kintsukuroi) on the Internet, and talk together about it …

Now, using the art materials here, I invite you to create an image of a cracked or broken bowl, chalice or piece of pottery …

Think about:

What do the cracks mean to you? …

Do they repel you, or invite attention? …

Then, fill in the cracks in whatever way/colour you choose, and as you do this, consider what the process of repair means to you. Think also of what kinds of actions and behaviour you might suggest to repair and cherish the 'cracks' in people experiencing mental ill health, in ways which include and respect the person's totally unique beauty …

Consider what societal measures may be represented by the precious 'filler', for example: good psychiatric support, consistent financial benefits, opportunities for meaningful daily activities …

Give folk a good amount of time to create their artwork and to reflect. Play some music during this, for example, 'Anthem', by Leonard Cohen, or 'Vincent', by Don McLean. Have some completed pieces of artwork placed around the worship space to give folk ideas, or have someone first demonstrate making a piece of art.

Sharing of artwork and insights:

Including the quotes:

'There is … a crack in everything
That's how the light gets in.'

Leonard Cohen, from the song 'Anthem', from *The Future*

'Blessed are the cracked – for the light can shine through them.'

Attributed to Groucho Marx[2]

You might want to do the sharing in small groups. Take your time; let everyone share their artwork and thoughts if they'd like to.

Song: 'All are welcome' (*Church Hymnary 4*, 198)

Scripture reading: Joel 2:28

*Then afterward
   I will pour out my spirit on all flesh;
your sons and your daughters shall prophesy,
   old people shall dream dreams,
   and young people shall see visions.*

Redeeming our cracks: liturgy 63

Reflection/Statement of intent:

We are accustomed, in reflecting on scripture, to honour and revere the gifts of prophecy, vision and the effects of the Spirit being *'poured out'*.

But in people deemed mentally ill, signs of similar occurrences will almost inevitably be subject to psychiatric diagnosis, medication, exclusion and often restraint.

Many people on psychiatric medication report a deadening of their spirit, their life-force, and a loss of creativity.

This can be a difficult area because some people deemed mentally ill do have delusions or hallucinations which may cause harm to themselves or others.

Thinking back to your reflections during the art meditation on what societal measures may be represented by the precious 'filler' in the cracks, I invite you now to identify one or two 'I will' statements of intent for yourself, and to write them on the strips of paper. For example: 'I will try to listen more to people', or 'I will help to campaign for better financial support for those experiencing mental health challenges.'…

When you're ready, and if you'd like, please come and place the strips of paper on the table in the crossing.

After folk are finished, have someone come and light the central candle on the table.

Prayer of intent:

This could be said by everyone.

Today, Lord, we have considered
our sisters and brothers,
and, of course, ourselves,
for in your eyes and in life,
we are not divided.

Yet we know that the world at large
would seek to keep us apart.

We know this is not your will –
and we seek to do your will:
by our statements of intent
to take action in the world.

So we ask for your blessing on our actions,
however small,
that joined together
we may create real change
in ourselves
and in the world.
Amen

Blessing

Recessional: 'We will take what you offer', from *There Is One Among Us*, John L Bell, Wild Goose Publications

Folk could take their artwork home, or it could be exhibited in the church, hall, etc.

You might have some information from a mental health charity, like Mind, available for people to take away with them.

Yvonne Morland

Sources and acknowledgements:

1. From 'Kintsugi: The Centuries-Old Art of Repairing Broken Pottery with Gold', by Kelly Richman-Abdou, from the website My Modern Met: https:mymodernmet.com/kintsugi-kintsukuroi. Used by permission of Kelly Richman-Abdou

2. For other quotes about brokenness and light see: https://quoteinvestigator.com/2016/11/16/light/

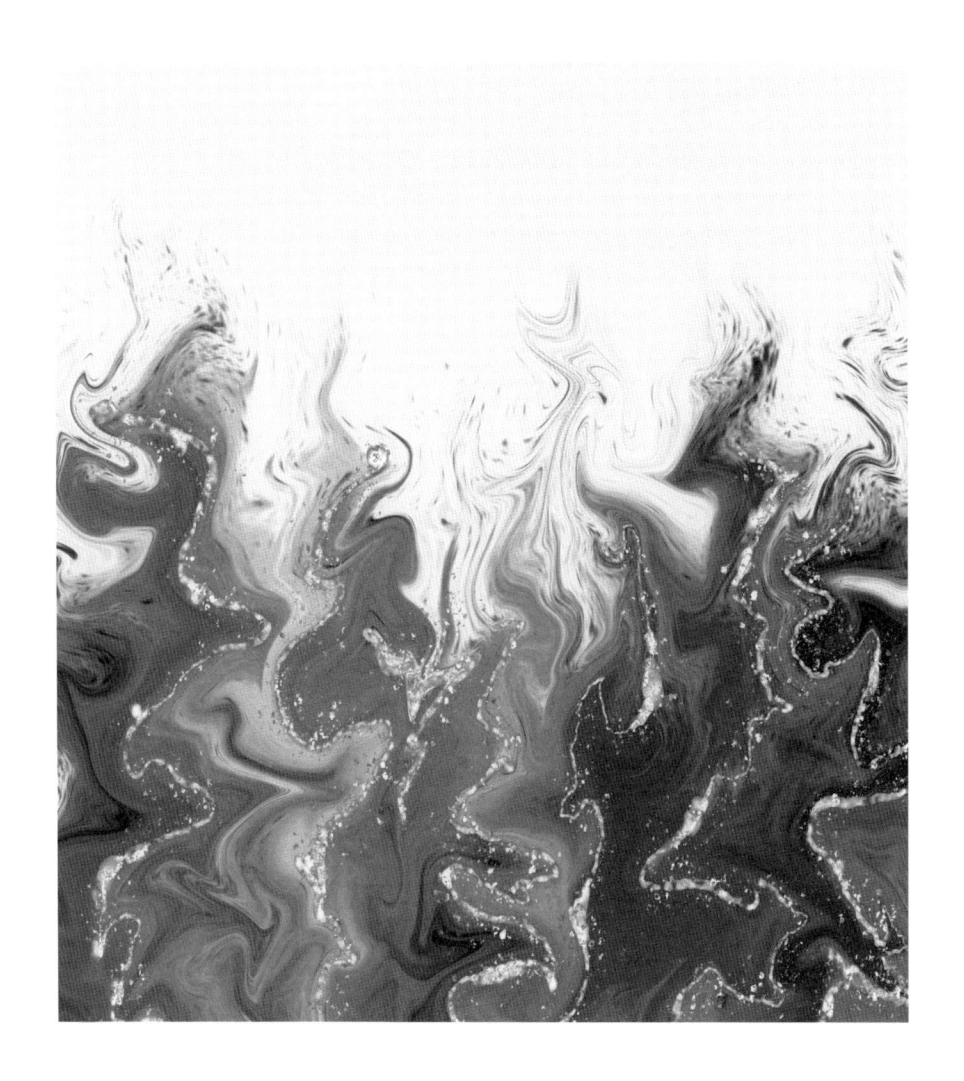

Poems

Write bravely, poems by Emma Major

I've got so many poems about mental health. Once I started gathering poems together by the mental health theme it was hard to stop. Some of these date back to 2004; some were written during the week I submitted them for this book.

– Emma Major

Depression

Dark
    Low
        Alone
            Cold

Unworthy
    Unnoticed
        Sad
            Anxious

Despairing
    Flat
        Grey
            Dull

No
    hope
        No
            point

Help
    Please
        Someone
            Please

I wear a mask

I wear a mask
On days like this
When life is hard
And I have to live
As if all's OK
And I'm coping fine
When actually
I'm falling off the line

So I put it on
And wear it all day
No one can see
I don't have to say
How I really feel
I'd be naked then
So I keep on going
Until I'm home again

Can you see me?

Turn around
Can you see
Through the pain
It's me?

Shield your eyes
Can you see
In the gloom
It's me?

Look closer
Can you see
Half-hidden
It's me?

Don't leave
Can you see

Almost broken
It's me?

Come back
Can you see
All alone
It's me?

Too late
Can you see
I'm gone
No more me?

Grey days

It's a grey day
With endless grey skies
It matches my low mood
Let me tell you why

The road seems endless
Constantly hemmed in
No light on the horizon
How's that to begin?

But over that fence
Are fields of wonder
With beauty living wild
To that I surrender

Despite the grey day
I'll find my sunlight
With friends around me
I know I'll be all right

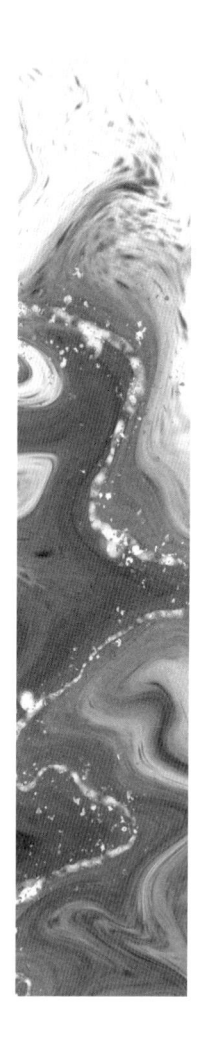

Rock-bottom dumps

What do I mean when I say I feel
Down in the rock-bottom dumps?
Am I a bit blue?
A little off colour?
Perhaps fed up?
Or do I mean something more?
Well, this time I meant a whole lot more
I meant a complete lack of desire to
Think
Eat
Move
And an overwhelming desire to
Sleep
Sleep deeply
Sleep deeply forever
That's what it's like for me
Hopefully not for too long.

Courage

Courage is standing up for the bullied
When everyone else turns their back

Courage is disagreeing with others
For what you believe in

Courage is not showing fear
So your kids don't panic

Courage is showing emotion
When everyone else clams up

Courage is just being you
Not trying to fit in

Courage is smiling
Even when you're hurting

Courage is asking for help
When you're trying to be strong

Courage is living

Gentle winds

Gentle winds
Calm anxious minds

Star sleeping
Soothes stressful souls

Fuchsia prayers
Brighten twilight friendships

Sunset blessings
Heal slippery apologies

Sea breezes
Refresh energy

Birdsong
Distracts pain

Sounds of nature
Connect with God

Cloud watching
Encourages peace

Wisdom

Stop often
Reflect and appreciate
Beauty every day

Do not judge yourself
Accept yourself as you are
You are amazing

Notice the beauty
The simple yet glorious
Miraculous

Know my peace

Come to me
With your worries and doubts
Leave them at my feet

Fear no more
What every new day brings
I'm your safe shore

Relax a while
Let my love surround you
Know my peace

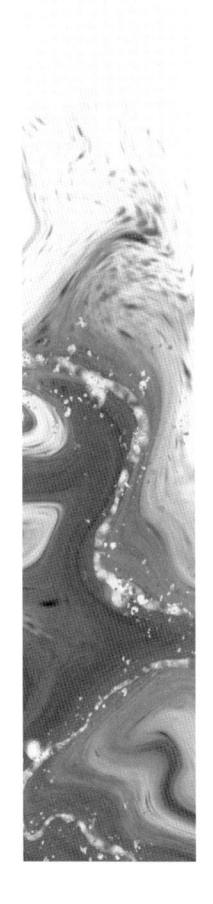

Eye of the storm

A month in a day
A week in an hour
Keeping positive
Then darkly dour

Through every change
Something to learn
With God's help
His anchor firm

Life's uncertainties
Sweep and whirl
Tornados of emotions
Swirl and curl

Eye of the storm
Faith retained
At the very centre
Hope obtained

Anxiety

Concern erupts
Worry builds
Heartbeat races
Fingers chill

Head pounds
Legs go weak
Tummy turns
I cannot speak

Feel sick
Might faint
Help please
All constrained

It's my heart
Got to get out
Want to move
I can't shout

Hand held
Words whispered
Eyes close
Voice whimpers

Help at hand
Calming slowly
Breathing better
Praying thanks to Holy

The horror is over
My voice is back
The body is working
Goodbye anxiety attack

Me, myself and I

I'm not that keen on me
Never ever really have been
It's ingrained, deep inside
Something about me I've tried to hide
But sometimes I need to share
What I am and how I care
About what it's like feeling this
And how it brings me to my knees
God has done much caring
Showing me that I'm worth loving
Slowly it's seeping through
But it's hard to remember when I'm blue

I never expect to be
Completely happy being me
But I hope that with God's love
I'll learn that I'm good enough

Surviving in the dark

For seven months I've been
Surviving in the dark
Every day a struggle
No light, no joy, no spark

Not wanting to get up
Not caring about much at all
Wishing it could be over
But trying hard not to fall

Celebrating small wins
Like getting out of bed
Fighting for perspective
Inside my heavy head

Searching for solutions
Trying anything I could
Battling the frustration
Of being misunderstood

Through all those endless weeks
I've never felt alone
God's been right beside me
His love I've always known

I can only imagine
How hard it would have been
Without support of church
And all the love within

Millions of people
Know this darkness in their lives
Don't know where to turn to
As they're trying to survive

It's time to make a difference
To talk about the pain
To break taboos around it
Eradicate the shame

Write bravely

Write bravely
Raise your voice
Share your mysteries
With God rejoice

Across peaceful lakes
Skim your stones
Float on air
Walk paths unknown

Don't bury hope
About what you wrote
Write letters, songs
Or just a note

Never be afraid
To share vulnerability
Delve within
Explore creativity

Peace descends

From our perspective
Chaos reigns
But step back
Take a God perspective
Beauty emerges
Through complexity
Diversity
Amidst pain and suffering
Truth appears
Peace descends
Light shines
Darkness ends

Emma Major

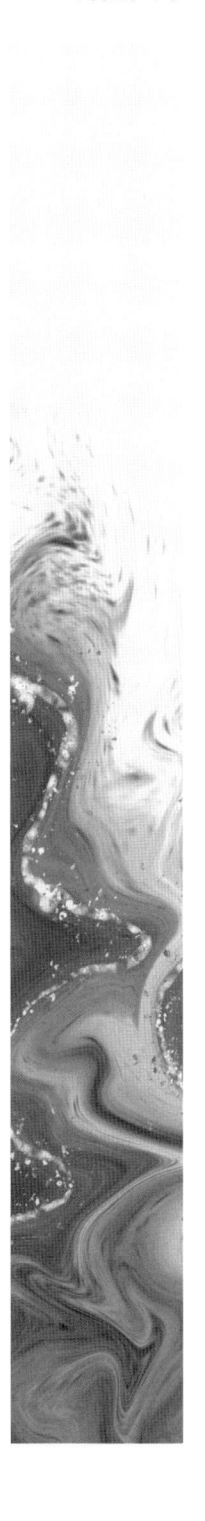

Pilgrimage, poems by Rosie Miles

You come here

*'Let us rid ourselves
of what we need to carry no longer'*
From the Iona Abbey Worship Book

You come here
   tired and aching
      weary of the life
         that weighs you down.

You come here
   vulnerable and hurting
      afraid of letting others
         touch your wounds.

You come here
   lonely and cynical
      finding it hard to praise
         the good world.

You come here
   and the thin places
      in your shell self
         start to crack open …

You come here
   and you are welcomed,
      included, given
         generous hospitality.

You come here
   and fresh-baked bread nourishes.
      In the carved cloister
         you find freedom, beauty.

You come here
   and you wrestle a blessing.

    You are not healed
        but forgiven.

You come here
  and the tomb around your heart
    breaks. Your salt tears
      mingle with the shore.

Good Friday

'We pray that you will teach us how to die …
But above all that you will teach us how to live.'

Said as part of the Good Friday liturgy in Iona Abbey, 25/03/16

The wind howls round the Abbey
like a kettle's shrill whistle.
The Sound is full of storm
and the bells ring at the wrong time.
All is out of joint.

This is the bitterest of days
but the rooks still build their nests
and the ferry will cross if it can.
A few people gather,
bracing themselves for the cold.

Beryl kneels. Stephanie sits on the floor.
Sally goes to the side chapel,
watches the sea. Nicola leaves.
Returns with a shawl to wrap round her legs.
Aidan stays near the back.

We are not here to be comforted.
We are here to mourn. All the pieces
of our selves which fear death
are here, listening to Christ's last words,
knowing the hour is near.

My sadness

I proffer my sadness
    You hint at gladness
I leave you my fear
    Its shadow is near
I offer my despair
    The wounds are still there
I give you my shame
    You say my name

Wound

Wound I do not want
Depths to which I will not descend
Risk I fear to take
    Forgive me

Loss I cannot bear
Shame I refuse to lose
Soul to which I won't listen
    Forgive me

May your brow be blessed

May your brow be blessed with soothing oil.
May its fragrance give you joy.
May its warmth comfort you.
May it be worked into your broken places
and may it light the lamp that shows you tomorrow.

Pilgrimage

I threw my shame
into St Columba's Bay.
This time it sank.

Instead I picked up
greenstone:
a small egg of hope.

That night my dreams
were full of girls
swimming.

Bethseda

Jesus said to the man at Bethesda
So do you really want to be well?
like he wasn't sure, he couldn't tell.

And you too: do you really want
to put down that rucksack of rocks
you've carried for so long, take them out

one by one and make a cairn? – a marker
to say you were here for a while, but
now you're moving on and

you've already divested yourself of
your bag your coat your shirt and
soon you're naked on the side of the pool.

Let the waters cleanse you. Feel
your fins bud in the echo of some greater
ocean, which whispers, caresses, shows you

how to live and move into this
new element. You're fish now free of all
that holds you. Pick up your mat. Walk.

Rosie Miles

Finding the fish, poems by Christine Dowling

Tribute to M

The world is a much duller place without her.
The funeral tribute in the paper said:
'A much-loved member of the community –
too loud not to be heard, too colourful not to be seen.'
She had been known to mental health services since she was 18
and it dominated most of her life.

Initially the cause of her sudden death was not known.
I remember a colleague coming to say to me:
'She would not have taken her life, not M – she loved life!'
And we found out she had not,
but the years of psychiatric medication
probably played their part.

Amidst her periods of lows she *did* love life –
and celebrated it to the full.
I only got to work with her for about one year;
she could at times be demanding and embarrassing
and on one occasion screamed in my face
that I was no fucking good to her.
But she also taught me lots about
childlike fun, appreciating life, thoughtfulness and kindness.

Her funeral was a fitting tribute.
We wore colourful clothes at the family's request.
Her coffin was painted with bright sunflowers.
You could tell her hand was in the songs
as we struggled to sing 'Amazing grace' alongside Elvis Presley,
before giving up and just letting the recording play.
I could imagine her looking down
smiling and laughing with affection.

I always feel that a fitting tribute to the ones
who come into our lives
and then go is:

If after their death you think of them
and it makes you smile
(not so with everyone)
then it is a fitting tribute.

M was one of those people.
And the world is definitely a much duller place without her.

I'm losing my mum to dementia

I'm losing my mum to dementia
and most of the time it is painful,
as day by day a bit more of the person I know slips away,
as I journey with her into the unknown.

'Remind me again what moussaka is,' she says,
as I explain with a pang that it is a Greek dish that she likes
and used to buy as a ready meal when she had the opportunity.

But my mum, who has never been demonstrative in worship,
came with me to my church yesterday
and sat there moving her hands
in an expression of her praise.
So with many losses come some gains.

When you feel vulnerable,
you have to trust.

When you don't understand,
you have to rely on those around you to explain
and to keep you safe.

When you cannot remember,
you discover things afresh,
like the taste of moussaka for the first time.

You see love on the dementia ward

You see the full range of emotions on the dementia ward.
But above all you see love.
Pure unconditional practical acted-out love.

Love from the wife who dutifully visits her husband,
wiping gently the dribble from his mouth.

Love from a partner who
after dancing with her husband
dances with another patient
so he does not feel left out.

Love in one patient helping another one up,
as he is unsteady on his feet.

Love in the two ladies who wander together
chattering away though no one,
not even each other,
appears to understand what they are saying.
But they know they are friends.

Love in the staff who
day to day
manage challenging situations and verbal and physical abuse.
From patients who are confused and frightened.
Who will
the next day
not remember
what was done or said.

Love in calming words and physical touch.

Love in searching out someone's favourite biscuit.

In the midst of the daily sadnesses and losses the illness causes.

You can see love on the dementia ward.
Pure unconditional practical acted-out love
day after day.

Finding the fish

He stopped by the lake in the park
as the rest of the group wandered on.
'I'm looking for fish,' he said.
I let out an inner sigh.
Then gently began to explain that
I didn't think he'd see any fish,
as an ornamental lake in a park was
too artificial and shallow.
But he was right and I was wrong,
I and the rest of the group.
As he pointed, I could see
two large sandy-coloured koi carp.

Later on, he stopped and pointed out more fish for us.
We would have missed them all
if he had not helped us to look.

We would have missed
small pieces of the wonder
and moments of calm.

Christine Dowling

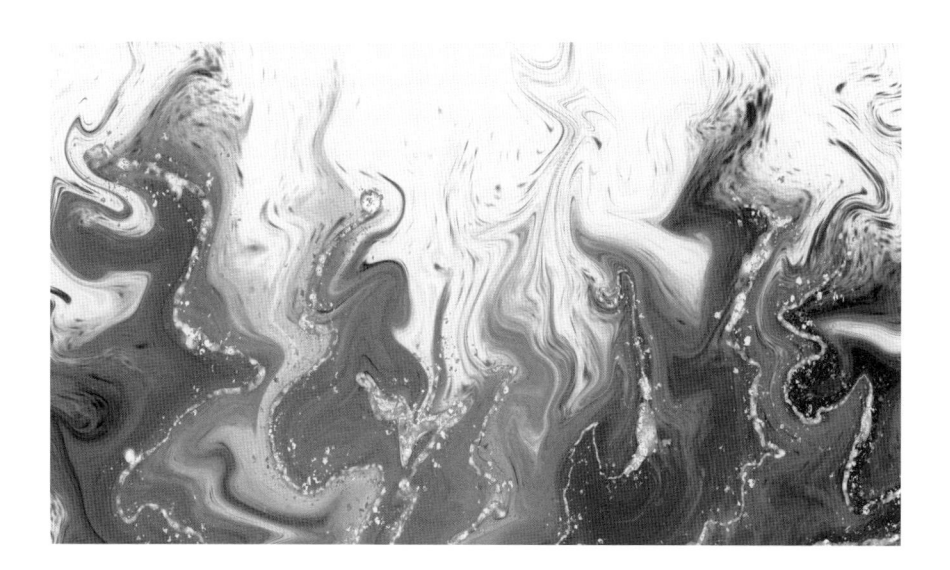

The day I lost my Mum, poems by Tricia Creamer

The day I lost my Mum

A bright new mug stood set for tea
which Mum, delighted, offered me.
'Granny gave it when she came,' she said.
'But she's been dead a while,' I said.
'Oh yes … yes. How silly!' she said.

I looked and heard; knew instant dread.
Realising life's a muddle,
seeking shelter in a cuddle,
I tucked her gently against my breast,
this sparrow falling from its nest.

Our comfort roles would now reverse –
my love would have to stretch and nurse.
'There's too much in my head,' she sighed.
My silent tears fell deep inside.

Family confusion

When Mum has lost and lost again
the way of life that makes it sane …
When her whole world is in a bag
and energetic spirit flags …
Sliding sideways to delusion,
making sudden weird allusions …
Then, the family she loves
are shocked in sad confusion.

They call for doctors, nurses, friends
to salvage and explain the bend
that swerves to raw exposure cold
leaving just her hands to hold.
They look for logic's safety route –
Mum chooses childhood substitute.
Her gobbledegook makes them smile
and weep, to see her so fragile.

When they chat about their mother,
recognise her in each other,
find genetic strength united
lifting fog to be clear-sighted –
a single fact looms from the gloom
opening like a gentle bloom –
her love which stretched across the years
will reach them now and stem their tears.

The week my mother lay dying

The snow lay deep, ice frozen hard,
sky wide open and blue;
trees standing still, waiting for spring …
the week my mother lay dying.

Daughters and sons rushed quickly home,
torn with comfort and care.
Grandchildren sadly saying farewell
to my mother, quietly dying.

Opening eyes she kissed a sweet smile
then slept to heal the end.
Knobbled hand squeezed a known hallo;
tender gifts at her dying.

Snowdrops appeared, crocuses bloomed,
tears slipped silently down.
Skiers away on the mountaintops
sent peace to my mother, dying.

Her bold bright spirit leaves her,
laughter and song soar high.
Blessed release to creation's fine hand;
new life at the birth of her dying.

My mother died of vascular dementia.

Clearing the papers

Papers, and Mum;
and papers.
Paperclips, pins, pennies.
Papers. Oh, Mum.

Little ducks, Christmas,
pots and boxes,
keys, scissors,
papers.

Bills, brochures, adverts, prayers,
years of diaries,
cards to send, cards received
in bags and boxes
of papers.

Big paintings,
precious china,
holiday gifts from every child
never tucked away,
placed with pride –
a knick-knack store;
and papers.

Gold and diamonds,
her husband's gifts,
her champion's prizes
the source of her private happiness;
and papers.

A kitchen, her hub,
too many clothes,
a shed full of wood,
Great Granny's bowl,
Great Grandpa's clock,
the carvings we witnessed;
and papers.

We select, share, decide.
Anxious for a piece to treasure;

anxious not to seem greedy;
anxious to show realism;
desperate not to break down
and cry: 'I want her! She's *mine*!'

Lost is she now,
as muddled as the skip
which now stands on the drive,
heaped with fragments of a life
she tried so hard to remember.
Bits of her discarded and gone.

Suddenly, almost unnoticed,
a surprise amongst the papers!
A lost treasure
more precious than everything,
found, smoothed,
tenderly held,
quietly declared:
her navy blue leather
searched-for
fish-studded
hymn book.

In this tightly tied bag,
stuffed with papers,
her soul is found
in lines
sung by heart and heaven
in a voice
rich with music and laughter.

She is alive,
will never die.
And we, her diligent children,
rescue, hold and honour her,
our Mum,
in this, our sad, tired task.

Tricia Creamer

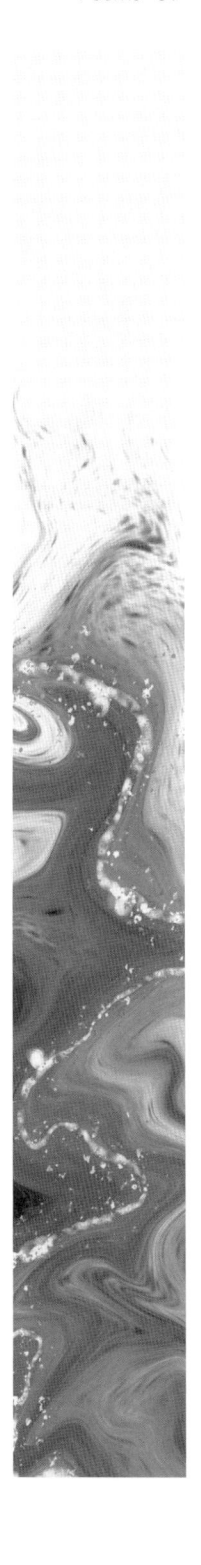

What is happiness?, poems by Janet Lees

One of those days

On those days when things seem to be
slipping from my grasp,
or I feel like hiding in a corner
unwilling to come out,
I hear you say:

'Plant a tree; sit under it',
and I think of us there,
under our tree,
laughing together.

But best of all,
I think of the one you said yesterday:
'Only dead fish go with the flow',
and I know it is so,
and I get ready to test my flanks against the current
and feel the oxygenated water
rushing through my gills
as I negotiate the rocks and rapids
and the swiping bear's paws,
as I leap up to the source of the river.

(It was my daughter Hannah, then a teenager, who said 'Plant a tree'.)

What is happiness?

To understand that
we need to consider
some of the things that count as unhappiness.
What makes us sad?

I am sad when my spirit seeps away,
when I mourn multiple losses,
both my own and those I carry for others.

I am sad when my pride is hurt,
when I feel thwarted, rejected,
unheard or cut off.

I am sad when there is no peace,
my dreams are haunted, sleep is hard to find,
the news is replete with disaster
and there is no sense of where to go next.

I am sad when I feel got at,
betrayed or attacked,
my judgement not valued
or my identity not affirmed.

Yes, insults can make me sad,
but it's mostly more subtle stuff
that heaps up and squeezes me
so that I can't think or speak without crying.

That's when I'm sad.

I am happy when justice is done,
and there is no further need to be angry,
which can be so exhausting.

I am happy when my identity is affirmed,
not lost in paragraphs of jargon
or bundled up in red tape.

I am happy when my voice is heard,
so that change can happen
and new life can flourish.

Lost

You can get lost in a temple
or anywhere at all.
You can wander about for a few days.
Or much, much longer.
Until the story comes back to you.
Then you remember
your place in God's kindom.
And you set off again,
firmer, clearer, resolved.

All cracked up (In Ampleforth Abbey)

There are cracks everywhere:
in the ceiling and the arches,
in the earth, in the institutions, in the people.

And our response to these cracks:
we keep Lent again.
We tell each story as if for the first time.
We count each encounter.

'Listen with the ear of your heart':
Benedict begins the Rule that way.
It's simple enough.

Jesus goes up a mountain.
Heaven breaks through.
There are cracks
but they can be filled with light and glory:
remember.

And then he comes down.
It is not the end of the story.
Even if it is a good reason for going up mountains,
it is not a good enough reason
never to come down again.

At the bottom of the mountain,
I am still drawn there,

to another encounter.
This one counts for me.
The excluded child and family;
feared and fearful.
Both faith and doubt need help:
both have their cracks.

The listening one listens
and another glory fills
the fragile lives of that family.

The story does not end there.
More cracks to come,
and more glory.

As the sun streamed into the Abbey church later,
many of the cracks were filled with
warm-coloured light from the windows.
Jesus: everything he's cracked up to be.

With arms open

Arms open, ready
to catch, to hold, to welcome:
arms open, face smiling.

Arms open,
you welcome;
you welcome me.

Arms open:
my mouth is open
in amazement.

Arms open:
there in the darkness
our arms are open.

Experience before Vespers, Ampleforth Abbey Crypt

Janet Lees

Note:

1. Some of these pieces are from Janet Lees' blog: https://foowr.org.uk/notesfrombambi

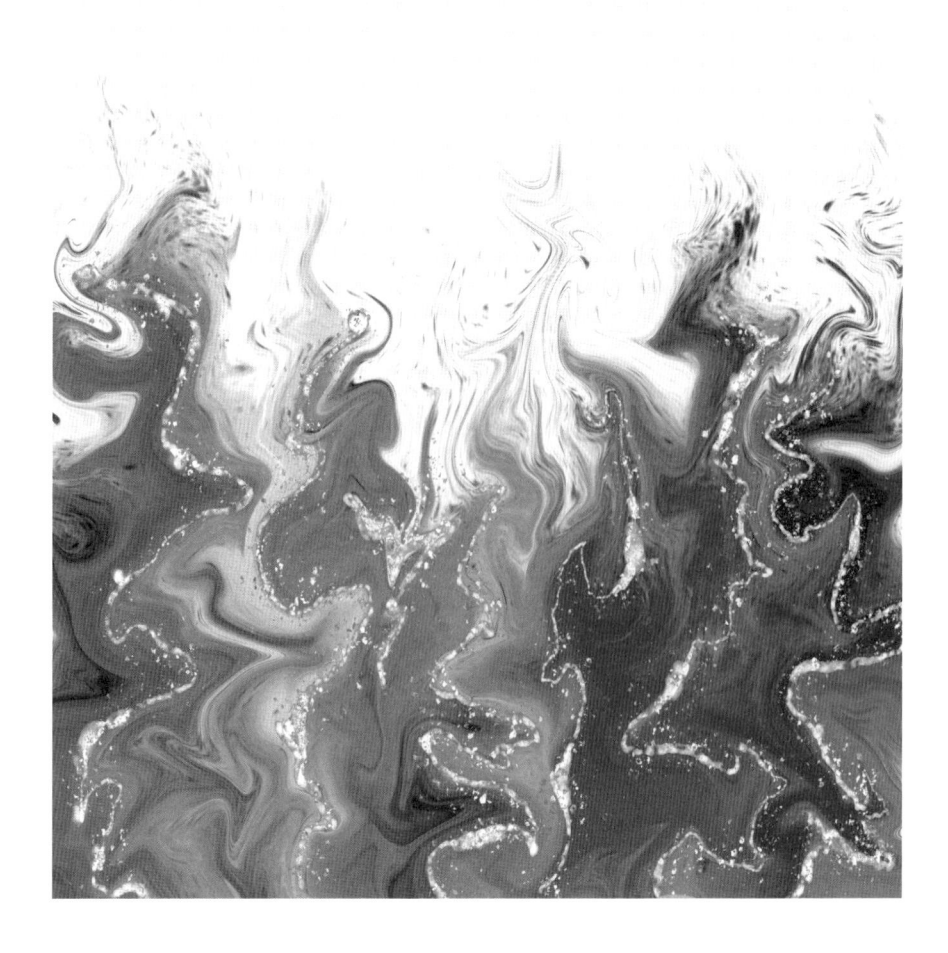

Bipolar story, poems by David Norman

Introduction:

My care through mental health services began in 1973. The symptoms I displayed, following a very meaningful spiritual emergence, were confused with psychotic symptoms, and pathologised.

My life became a matter of dealing with successive ups and downs.

At a retreat in the mid-1990s I was introduced to Rublev's icon of the Holy Trinity, also known as The Hospitality of Abraham. *Rublev drew his inspiration from the story in Genesis of the three strangers visiting Abraham. This icon touched me deeply, expressing the mutual, unconditional love that the Three Persons of the Trinity have for each other, and into which we are all drawn to share. I wrote a poem during the retreat about what it meant to me.*

Not long afterward, while in one of my dark, down moods, I wrote a poem that connected my feelings with those of Jacob, when he wrestled with a man at Peniel (Gen 32:22–31). As I look back at these poems I realise that they have kept me going, giving me hope in the dark times.

While working with a clinical psychologist, and with a transpersonal counsellor, I was encouraged to express myself in painting, as I had done from time to time in the past. Painting then led me to writing more poems. Most of them are just little rhymes, but some have more of a narrative style. Through all this I have kept in mind the mental health services' concept of 'recovery' and the Christian understanding of 'healing'.

In mental health practice, 'recovery' is understood as a process, a journey, during which a mental health service-user learns to live life as fully as possible, in spite of symptoms remaining.

A wise, elderly Anglican priest, who has been much involved in the healing ministry, explained to me during another retreat that 'healing', in the Christian sense, is about living life as fully as possible even though there is not a physical 'cure'. (My wife has progressive multiple sclerosis and is totally dependent on me for her care; she is confined to a wheelchair, needs help with toileting and showering, needs hoisting for all transfers, cannot prepare her own meals; but there is something that shines out of her which makes me feel she is the most 'healed' person I know.)

The similarities between these two understandings, 'recovery' and 'healing', is worth considering, and taking to heart. I think they lie behind my own search, my own journey.

The poems I have written recently have tumbled out as ideas come to mind and I reflect on them. I feel that they are saying something to me to enable me to normalise, and cope with, life in a more positive way, as it unfolds. I share some of them here, as they may be helpful to others and encourage them to express some of their own hidden feelings, perhaps in poetry, prose or painting, and so find a way forward on their own journeys.

– David Norman

Meditation on the Trinity

On Rublev's icon of the Holy Trinity

Be still and know:
    that I am God: Father, Spirit, Son.
Be still and know:
    the Son's Friendship, the Spirit's Help, the Father's Trust.
Be still and know:
    the Son's Compassion, the Spirit's Counsel, the Father's Wisdom.
Be still and know:
    the Son's Strength, the Spirit's Fire, the Father's Power.
Be still and know:
    the Son's Peace, the Spirit's Truth, the Father's Justice.
Be still and know:
    the Son's Faith, the Spirit's Hope, the Father's Glory.
Be still and know:
    the Son's Service, the Spirit's Guidance, the Father's Majesty.
Be still and know:
    the Son's Love, the Spirit's Grace, the Father's Might.
Be still and know:
    the Son's Closeness,
        the Spirit's Freedom,
            the Father's Infinite Otherness.

Be still and know:
    Forgiveness by the Son,
        Adoption by the Spirit,
            Reconciliation with the Father.
Be still and know the Son.
Be still and know the Spirit.
Be still and know the Father.
Be still and know the Lord,
    the Three-in-One.
Be still and know Him,
    the Wonder, the Joy, the Pain.
Be still and know,
be still,
be,
and know my Self,
    at one with Him.

Bipolar story

Risen, ascended Lord in glory
pictured in the high clerestory.
I heard your voice from there above.
It told me of your heavenly love.
What joy, what overwhelming joy,
I felt again like some young boy
who, looking from a mountaintop,
must halt his walking and take stock
of all the wonder he can see,
and know that he can be, just be.
It is in be-ing he's set free.

The doctors thought that I was mad
and gave me all the drugs they had;
but these turned out to be a curse
because I ended so much worse.
They sent me back to teach my classes,
my mind a blur, just like my glasses.
On drugs I could not think, or function,

recall the facts that need a mention.
And so I failed to keep much order;
my pupils just seemed to take over.
Classified 'unfit to teach'
I lost the job I'd strived to reach.
In darkness now, like down a well,
I felt I really was in Hell.

I could not stay here, God-forsaken.
What could I do, now out of action?
Without an income we'd all starve –
how could we keep ourselves alive?
The only thing that I could do
was to retrain, start out anew.
Foot set, again, upon the ladder,
I learned accounting needs an adder.
I found a post in new employment;
it had not quite the same enjoyment
I'd had when, as a young fit teacher,
my pupils opened like an oyster.

Then, after years at office desk,
I thought 'I really need a rest
from spreadsheets, budgets and from ledgers,
quarter's figures on computers!'
Return to the classroom would be fine.
Now well again, and in my prime,
I found a post that fitted well.
I had returned from death and Hell.
This led me on to seek and find
another post I had in mind,
to see me through to my retirement
when I had finished all employment.

It's been a life of ups and downs;
I've yet to find the smoother plains.
Perhaps all life is just like that:
it's never really, really flat.
'*Carpe diem*', seize the day,
this really is the only way.

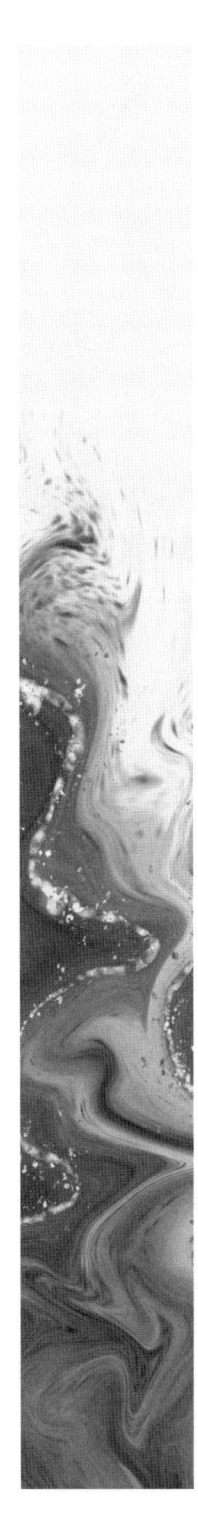

Love

I'm knocking at your door to say
I love you: I will love you always.
I bring my light into your life;
lift you from sadness, darkness, strife.
Listen to me;
lend me your ear.
I'll heal your wounds, at cost so dear.

Yes, there is healing in my touch;
healing and wholeness, love and trust.
No need to fear
for I am near;
I'm ever close,
just at your rear.

You'll hear my voice behind you say,
'This is the way; a narrow way,
to tread with care,
and not to stray
to left or right;
but
carry on this way I show
'till all is done'.

The rocky boat

I stepped out of the rocking boat
and found I didn't sink but float.
Then panic!
I began to doubt,
for white-topped waves were all about.

But there's a figure, not on board.
I cry to Him. 'O save me, Lord!'
He reaches out His hand to me,
and plucks me from the raging sea.

We join the others – all astounded
that faith in Him proves not unfounded.
'Why did you doubt? O little faith,
it's really me, it's not a wraith.
For I am always ever near.
Trust me to calm you when you fear.'

Found

What is there now to do or say?
I went for a walk just yesterday,
to lay the ghost of things now past,
to look ahead – at last, at last.

We walked along, my friend and me;
a friend, or Friend, which could it be?
We walked along the paths again
that I had walked, sometimes in pain.

The pain with which my brother struggled,
and I myself, like Jacob, wrestled.
But something new caught my attention:
'Forget the past, give it no mention.'

The past is gone, like crops that grew
in fields we passed, admired the view.
The view was not of Crosby shore,
nor yet the fell I knew before.

For what I now could really see
was fields and fields surrounding me.
Fields that stretched to the horizon –
and arching skies that gave new vision.

My eyes seemed opened; as I viewed
I felt my hope had been renewed.
Hope of a future stretched before,
was here before me, at my door.

My friend, my Friend, my unseen Friend
was here to see me to the end;
the end of all my exploration,
giving me His full attention.

I'd sought for Him in many ways,
the search had occupied my days.
If I had stopped, just for a while,
I maybe would have sensed Him smile;
for He Himself had searched for me,
to find me and to set me free.

Now free at last to live each moment,
live it fully free from torment,
free from things now past, and gone,
to face the future, sing a song
of thankfulness and praise,
for all His mercy through my days.

David Norman

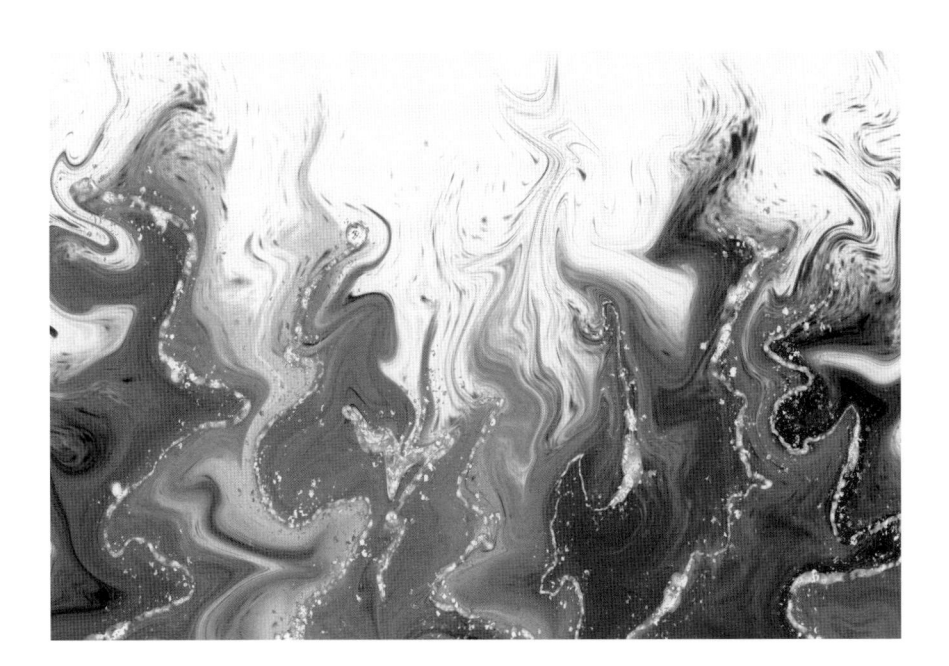

Craftswoman, poems by Bev Robertson

The lost message

I am not in the Temple
or the book.

I am not in the creed
or the ritual.

I am the breath of the breeze
the warmth of the sun
the roar of the sea.

I am.

Do not seek me in memories
or search for me in fears.

Do not find me in strategies
or teach of me in boundaries.

I am
as free as the birds
as wild as the beasts
as liquid as the dew.
I am you.

Craftswoman

So often I sit in the small room of my mind
knitting myself into the stitches of time.
Wondering and worrying about tomorrow,
angry and sad about yesterday.
You call to me to let go:
Give thought no more mind, you say.
Come here now and see.

So I lay down my needles of niggles
and put away my patchwork of predictions,
leave behind the looms of thought
and I sit on the cushion of
this moment.
And I breathe you in, filling my being,
and I breathe you out, smiling.

Now I am here and I see
the warp and weft of your world
bright-filled with you.
Light against dark and dark against light,
shape-shifting to form and freedom of line.
A painterly palette filled with
a multitude of greens and blue in leaf and sky,
distance and foreground,
and the light sparkling through it all.

Now I can return to my needles, my palette and paint
and join anew in the art of life
in all its fullness of curves and contrasts,
where even the darkness isn't dark any more,
it merely lends depth to the brightness
and richness to the raw material.

Bev Robertson

Some more poems

Homage to young men

'Homage to Young Men' was inspired by the GalGael Trust in Govan and first performed by me in January 2006 in King Tut's Wah Wah Hut, Glasgow, with the chart-topping duo Nizlopi (of JCB Song fame). This was released on the band's autumn 2006 album, and I am grateful to the lead singer, Luke Concannon, for permission to reproduce his chorus. (Alastair McIntosh)

I want to talk to all the young men out there
It's for the women too, but especially the men,
    'cos it's tough to be a young man in this world
You have to face so much heartbreak and loss
In love and career and life
It's easy to forget the meaning and give up
To burn up or sell out to addictions, despair or greed
Easy to forget that life's a journey
    with a beginning, a middle and an end
It's about navigating the future, your future
It's about learning to become a man who's real,
    and able to love

Are you waiting for me?
Are your hands down in the dirt?
We belong together
I've been longing since my birth
To be arms around you
To be true to who we are
To let all our pain out
To be playing in your heart

So let's talk about the first stage of life
The departure, when your boat is pushed out on the river
Most of who you are is still your small self
The you your family has made you,
    your schooling and your friends

You've still not found your deep self, your Great Self,
    'cos that's what the journey's for
So you set out, full of hope, but with a heavy load
All the baggage of your upbringing
All the love, yes, but the fucked-up-ness too
Maybe the absent father, or the smothering mother,
    or the cold indifference of those around you
It's no wonder you've a rough ride coming
It's gonna get tough and it's got to
So you can find your Self
So you can become, a real man

And that's when you hit the second stage of life
The initiation in the rapids and the storms
That's when you find the pain of brokenheartedness
Love affairs that fail, failures in career
    and all your hopes for what the world might have been
Plenty young men founder grazed on such jagged rocks as these
Bruised and angry in a storm of violence towards self and others
But it doesn't have to stay like that
No, my friends, not if you push on and open to the inner grace
    that will bring you courage
The courage to face reality as it is,
    without lies
The courage to know your wound but to outgrow it
    and insist on beauty
The courage to open your heart,
    to hold fast to truth,
        and to stand each step in dignity

And that's the courage that brings your boat to the third stage
    of life
To see how your small self is held in a greater Self
And that you're fit to be an elder in your community,
    able to share the gifts and the blessings
Able to support and inspire what gives life among your people
And to love your beloved,
    to love and be loved by the Beloved no less, my friends

Because we're talking here of love in all its meanings
And you can only love with a deepening heart
And that is why you had to grow courage on this journey to
    the ocean
That's what your battle wounds on the field of life were all
    about
That, my dear friends,
    is what qualifies you
        to be a man in your community
Capable of loving and able to be loved …
Capable of loving
and able to be loved …
Capable of loving
    and able
        to be
           loved

Alastair McIntosh

Receiving (A poem for John)

This poem was written twenty years ago when I worked at Camas, the Iona Community's Centre on the Isle of Mull. A closeness to nature and sense of community creates a nurturing environment at Camas. It offers a safe and sacred space for stories to be shared. For people who struggle with mental health, Camas often seems to bring a sense of peace and belonging, even after just a short time.

John (not his real name) came to Camas with a homelessness project. I had been very busy, and was worried I wouldn't have the energy to be fully present to our guests, something which was important to me. Listening to John was a privilege, and a gift. He told me his story of life in the army, followed by a breakdown and the loss of relationships at work and home. It was also a story of hope – of the courage he had to survive; of his creativity and skill, particularly in woodwork; of his compassion and desire to help others in similar situations.

The conversation with John was a place of grace, and reminded me that we are all gifted and flawed, all strong and weak, all able to teach and learn, to give and receive. This is part of the joy and challenge of being human. (Rachel McCann, a former Camas Coordinator)

Shyly showing me your smile,
slowly sharing your heart, your hope,
as close to you as the lifeblood
and as precious as the air.

I hold it in my hands,
anxious I may drop it, crack it, or even crush it
with clumsy words and tired mind.

I listen …
the poetry of your passion
leads me through the landscape of your dreams.
And I know you will go there – waking to see, as I see,
your strength in world-worn eyes,
your tenderness in work-torn hands.

I listen …
above the clamouring voices,
sometimes religiosity,
above demands and worries
that today feel heavy on me;
you whisper of the Mystery –
the leaves who are your sanctuary,
the stones who keep your soul.

I listen …
and with what you risk to give me,
I am renewed.

Rachel McCann

For information about Camas, see the Iona Community's website: www.iona.org.uk

A poem by Glyn

I met Glyn (not his real name) when I was working in a shelter for homeless men. Glyn was in his early 20s and waiting to get on the housing list. He spent his days in the public library, where it was safe and warm, drawing and reading and writing poetry. Glyn was shy and quiet, and cautious, but sometimes shared his poems with me. I sometimes wonder what happened to Glyn – he had such potential. (Ed.)

Depression

Morning …
feel it
enter my being …

Like cold rain
seeping
into a poorly constructed building.

Glyn

Depression

I stood alone
On the empty stage
The theatre had closed hours ago
The darkness was thick and tangible
And the silence crushed my thoughts

And in the corners of the darkness
The shadows stirred
I felt them start to move
Huge, black, towering shapes
Unseen in the blind night around
But I knew that they were closing in
Threatening me
Suffocating me
I knew them
And I was afraid

The first one enveloped me
And I recoiled in self-pity
Hated its presence
Wanted to destroy it
And its voice inside my head
Said,
'I am Pain'
And I was afraid

Another sucked itself into my lungs
It burst my screams into the silence
But I heard no answer
I mourned
And it breathed its name into me
And said,
'I am Grief'
And I was afraid

A third crept into my bowels
Gripped me and dragged me below a bottomless abyss
Below feeling
Into nothing
And its name bled into me
And said,
'I am Despair'
And I was afraid

And I knew that another possessed me
Froze me
Burnt me
Controlled me
And its name was Fear
And I was afraid

And around these moved others
Thick and dank and black
I knew them
And felt them
Hunger

War
Disease
Hate
And I belonged to them

And towards me came the last shadow
I looked into the black hole at its centre
And as I saw Death
I heard a voice that was mine, saying
'There is no God
There is no God
You don't exist'

And as I fell into that black hole
I heard a voice
Distantly
From the wings
A million light years away
Say,
'Yes I do
I do exist'

And there was nothing

I stood alone
On the empty stage
The theatre had closed hours ago
The darkness was thick and tangible
And the silence crushed my thoughts

And in the corners of the darkness
The shadows stirred
The first one moved towards me
And I looked at it
Knew it
Touched it
And felt Pain
And knew that it was mine
But knew too that I was Loved
And I was not afraid

Another came nearer
And I knew Grief
Knew that it was part of me
But as it saw that I knew Laughter
Felt Joy
And was not afraid
It shrank and could not hold me

And then I turned to face Despair
I saw it
Knew it
And it could not possess me
For I had found Hope
And I was not afraid

And yet I knew Fear
It was there
I held it
I felt it
But I was no longer afraid of it

And I could see the bottom of the black hole now
And it was filling up
With Life
Which would make it overflow
And drown Hunger
And drown Hate
And drown War and Disease
And drown Grief and Despair and Pain and Fear
With Life

And as the shadows shrank and aged
And I held them
And knew that they were mine
Not I theirs
I realised that I was not alone
Someone was standing in the wings
But I had forgotten to give the cue

And I realised that the lights had started to come up
And I remembered the cue
And whispered
'Yes,
You do
You do exist'

And you held me

Linda Hill

Names matter

Names are important.
We don't want to be known by our mental state or diagnosis:
anxious, sad, depressed, bipolar …
We want to be known by our name.

Names matter.
When someone knows our name
we know they have taken the trouble
to begin to know us.

When someone calls us by name,
there is a connection between us:
knowing one another's name is the beginning of relationship.

Relating to those who use our name
is the gateway to deeper fellowship,
is the road to stronger friendship.

In connecting with those
to whom our names matter
we find companionship and joy.

On the path to well-being
names matter.

Simon Taylor

Gerry

People called you

lazy
weak
a loser
fucked in the head

I used to think
if you were missing an arm or a leg
if you had been hit by a car
or had come back from a war
if you had a disease like cancer

they would have felt sorry for you
they would have looked on you as a hero
They would have been more forgiving of you
sittin' there on a bar stool all day long
drinkin' their hard-earned taxes.
They would have bought you a beer
(Sometimes they did buy you a drink

when they were feeling superior and generous,
during lulls in real life when they came slumming,
when they needed to stand beside you in order to get
a taller measure of themselves.

When they were down
and needed some understanding

Besides
you were a good drunk
You were harmless)

Gerry

you lived down the street
with your mom and dad
'Forty-three years old and still
living with his parents'

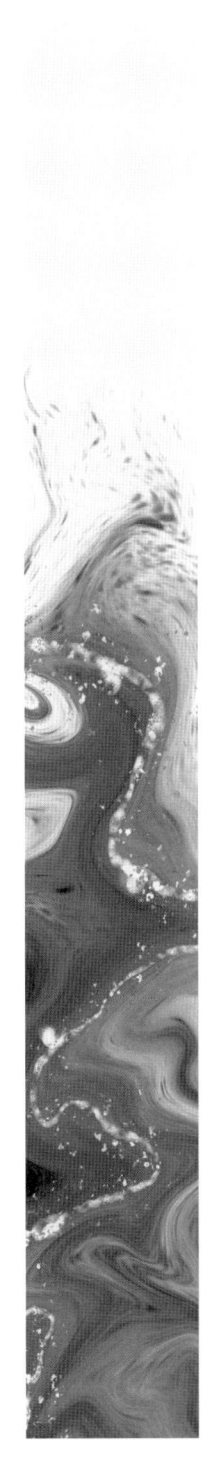

You never said much
but when I was growing up you lent me record albums:
Paul Simon's *Still Crazy After All These Years*
Imagine by John Lennon

They said a lot.

One day
you took me into your father's dark shed
which smelled of gasoline and grass clippings
(you cut lawns sometimes, did odd jobs)
and showed me your wood carvings:

a timber wolf
a Canada goose
an old man with a cane
the soul-lined face of a Native American woman

sculpted from pieces of driftwood you collected and
branches broken in storms
Sunlight came streaming in through the single window
and I saw you in a different light
You looked transformed
ascetic

Your work was beautiful and skilful

I said you should sell some
You said you didn't want to sell them. They weren't that good
'They *are* good,' I said

You smiled
and looked satisfied for a moment
happy

When I was a bit older
I used to see you
down at the Dominion Tavern on Saturday nights
You stayed over on 'the dead side',
with veterans sitting alone at sticky tables
and other old people

life had passed by and
left tangled in cobwebs

Sometimes I'd come over and talk to you

Once
on your birthday
you gave me some advice:
'Don't grow up like me,' you said –
and looked me in the eye

'Ah, come on,' I said
'Come on'

I wanted to get back to the music and lights
back to my friends
(back to 'the land of the living')
Everybody was there
The Bar Flies were playing
Layla Tajanii was dancing
in the close, summer heat

I stayed a little longer
and left an empty bottle beside you on the bar
I'd come back later to make sure you got home all right
I told myself
When I remembered
you were gone

Gerry

I heard you killed yourself

Slit your wrists in a park one night

(Someone walking their dog found you)

Ray the bartender told me when I came back to town one year
I ran into him walking down by the river
The Dominion was a steakhouse now
'Christ, I felt sorry for the kid,' he said

'Did anyone keep his wood carvings?' I asked
'His what?' he said

Gerry

I wish I could have said something to make you believe
you weren't a failure in life

Gerry

you touched me –
I wish I could have told you that
Would it have been enough?

I doubt it
I'm sure it wouldn't have. It never is

Gerry

I think you were heroic
to try to transform your pain

Strong
to have lasted as long as you did

Gerry

this world is crazy
can't see
the beauty
in brokenness

Neil Paynter

Anathema (ἀνάθεμα)

Unclean, unsaved –
leper bells might ring.
Dutiful, in charity,
the chosen few will sing,
protected by the wall of Mother Church.

Imperfect, unshriven –
damned by your own decree,
you, me,
whoever it might be:
are we accursed
or a gift offered to God?

Pamela Turner

It was easy for you

You were in a bad place.
You had been there for a long time,
there was no change.
You wanted change.
This seemed a way out.
A possibility of ending the pain.

But easy for you
was not easy for me.
I could not see inside your head.
See the wheels of reason
weighed down by sacks of clay
deadened by downward spirals
and darkened by clouds of despair.

It was not easy for me
to find you after,
to see what remained of what had been you.
Your pain extinguished
but mine just begun
pain of misunderstanding
pain of helplessness
pain of regret
pain of 'if only'
pain of never knowing why.

It was easy for you
but you have gifted me your pain.

John Butterfield

When I have lost my song (Matt 6:25–34)

Birds, come,
fly and sing to me,
when I have lost my song.

Trees, come,
and wave a branch to me,
when I feel alone.

Flowers, come,
pour your scent my way,
when I have lost my senses

and I will tiptoe
through my valleys
into a new tomorrow.

Elizabeth Baxter

The hollow

I

It was the hollowed-out
fossil-powered stone canoe
which was our nest. Childhood
drowned as we floated, sis
and I navigating and steering,
carrying our captains as we
carried their responsibilities

II

When really tiny, sis and I,
preschool both: Mum would
go wandering in Worksop
streets, by the canal, fields,
we knew not where, but feared:
frightened she'd never come back,
terrified she would.

She'd threatened to kill us.
We believed her.
She tried once, with me,
failed, thanks to the dog,
who deflected her aim
(he knew what she was up to)
so I landed on the sofa
instead of through the window.

She flew higher than space,
eagles could never reach her;
not even at Christmas
or one of our birthdays
when it was right
for kids to be at excess
could we match her height,
or she'd dive so deep
we could not fathom.

III

Grown up, Sis becomes a nurse
and I a social worker.

She gets the surgical prize,
stitches people back together.

Day-duty 1972
well-dressed siblings
aged eight and ten, boy and girl,
dumped at Collier Row, Romford,
Social Services Office, parents
pretend to be parking car
never return. I'm qualified then,
my hollowed-out self more useful;
it reaches their hurt where mine is;
we find Children's Home places.
It feels like nothing but it is care.

IV

The canoe nuzzles
into the ocean
preparing for
highs or lows
and nothings.

Robert Shooter

Under the comet

In 1997 (the year of the Hale-Bopp comet) my mother Edie (consistently called Alice by the authorities because that was her first name) was admitted to a psychiatric ward in the first stages of Alzheimer's disease. This poem reflects something of my daily visits to that (as it seemed to me) bleak, soulless place where helpers with limited training tried to cope with a milling crowd of men and women in varying stages of dementia.

Fortunately the last years of Edie's long life were spent in the tranquil surroundings of one of the superb specialist homes run by the Augustinian Order of nuns, but it is the vision of that grey, unforgiving ward (now demolished) that returns from the past to haunt my imagination.

Florence, Rose and Alice strut
   the ward's grey catwalk
   in relentless pursuit of freedom.
In the crook of Florence's arm
   is a bear with a bagged head –
   proof against toy thieves.

Rose chassés between her sticks
   as the gramophone spins
   her latest cha cha pupil
   up the linoleum street
   to where the locked door
   (PLEASE RING FOR ADMITTANCE)
   keeps the world at bay.

Alice fingers her dressing gown
  (ALL GARMENTS MUST BE CLEARLY MARKED)
  and eyes the bowling green
  through the Sluice Room window.
Another rink will soon be ending
  and, with more teas to prepare,
  she hurries to the kitchen.

Was it today that lunch came round
  two minutes since or
  when they lived at home and
  mother called them in from play?
Listen – she's calling now, and
  they must turn and tread
  the grey linoleum once more.

Upon the dayroom wall
  the season's written out with
  weather, date and menus
  brightly spread.
Just like those pictures
  on the classroom wall.
Is that today or
  sixty years ago?

The words are Wash and
  Toilet and Injection.
But what of Faith and
  Hope and Love?
How can they find
  the meaning of rejection
  when cells that gave that
  meaning life are gone?

Light years above the Sluice Room door
  Hale-Bopp shines on;
  predictable, remote.
Behind its forked tail
  Florence, Rose and Alice

strut the Milky Way,
curlers and stardust in their hair,
into a brighter dawn,
a farther shore,
where bears range free
and dancers spin
and every wood that's bowled
touches the jack.

Peter Charles Jackson

This poem took second place in the Alzheimer's Society's national competition for poems on dementia in 2009.

Myself

(Written following a breakdown, 2016)

I haven't been myself
lately, I said.
Who is this self
I haven't been?
Is it my prideful self
craving recognition,
intolerant of criticism?
Is it the self which
feigns compassion,
the pretending,
posturing,
judgemental,
resentful self?
The self which
after all these years
I hardly know
and fear to face?

Or is it the self
I deep down long to be?
The seed of which was

planted at my making?
And yet …
I am not a split person.
Myself is the whole of me.
The self I despise
and the self I long for
are not separate.
I cannot embrace one
and disown the other.
Can I deeply believe that
there is no particle of my being
that is despised or beyond
the reach of that love which
remains when all else is gone?

Warren Bardsley

Watching the duck

She sits at the water's edge
watching a duck float over the waves
in a gentle and relaxed rhythm.
Then it is suddenly submerged in rising waves.
It takes a dive into the deep waters
but soon resurfaces,
confident in its strength to deal with
this darkness,
and continues on its journey.

Watching the duck, she wonders
if her faith can bring her through
the deep waters she is facing:
depression, lack of motivation …
Maybe she can surface again and
again from this suffering,
safe in the knowledge that the gentle rhythm
will return in her life.

Katherine Rennie

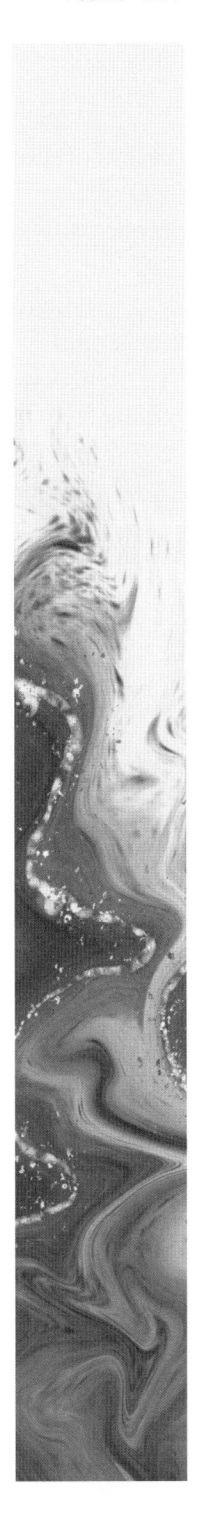

Fumbling forward

      Won't fumble
(backward) but forward. Might teeter, may totter,
(will) splatter paint onto the floor. Wear garish
purple that won't match the furniture. Curve UP
then
      down
then loop back loop back (looping).
      This is no U-turn but a spiraling down, not retreat
but dance.
      You won't be a lady.
      You'll be spectacular.

Jessica Wachter

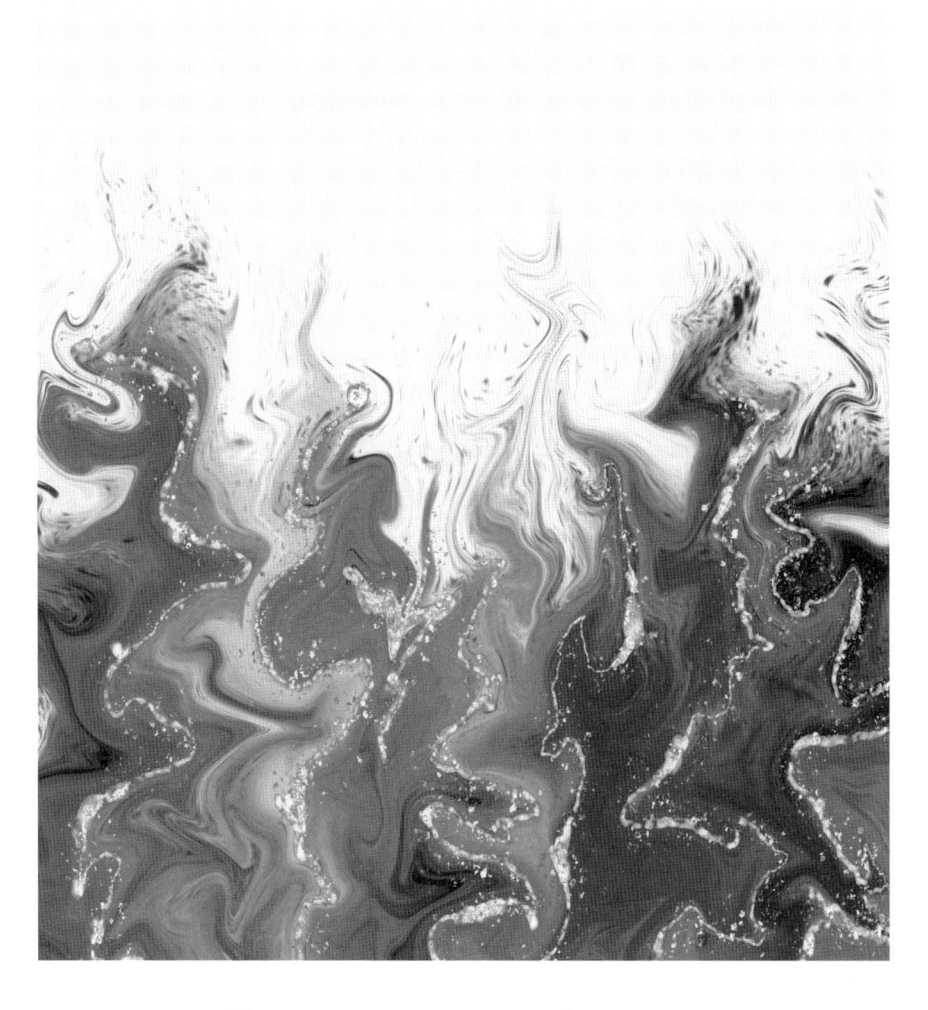

Reflections and stories

Personal stories

Spiritual emergency: Reflections of a mental health service user

There have been many changes in mental health care since the time, more than forty-five years ago, when I first had the need to be a user of mental health services. The change that most affects me is in the way in which my local mental health Trust integrates spiritual care with the medical care it provides; a change that has taken place in many other trusts too.

I was made aware in recent conversations with my Trust's chaplain, who is also the Manager of a Spiritual Care team within the Trust, that I could expect very different treatment now, in regard to my spiritual concerns, from that which I received in the crisis of 1973 and the years immediately following.

If I should become mentally unwell now, and have spiritual concerns and questions which I feel need addressing, then I can ask to meet with the chaplain, or one of his team, for pastoral help and guidance. Furthermore, while relatively well and living in 'recovery', I can prepare an Advance Statement, a legal document, to make sure that my spiritual care is not compromised or neglected in any treatment I receive from Mental Health Services, should that become necessary in the future. Also, any concerns of my near relative, in this case my wife, would be taken into account in designing my treatment plan. This is all a big change from what happened to me at the onset of my illness, when there was no chaplain, and I welcome it.

It all began in 1973. I was under pressure, as I was overseeing major building work both at home and at school (where I was a senior teacher), when my brother became mentally ill and was sectioned. I felt guilty that I had not foreseen this: I felt I should have helped him more. Still worrying about this, and in quite a state of anxiety, I went to evensong with my family, and during the first hymn heard a loud voice shouting out above the sound of the singing: 'Jesus is the Answer.' I soon realised that, surprisingly, nobody else had heard this voice, and concluded it had just been 'in my head'. However, there was an immediate change in my belief system, particularly in my beliefs about Jesus.

I was completely overwhelmed, and became confused and disoriented. This state didn't subside, so two days later my wife called our GP. He prescribed a powerful antipsychotic drug, which knocked me out for the next couple of days, after which he brought a psychiatrist to see me. As I made some sort of recovery I struggled back to school just before the end of term, in a very anxious state. I also had a follow-up appointment with the psychiatrist at the Mental Health Unit.

I was not given a diagnosis, but it was soon clear that the psychiatrist saw the 'voice in my head' as a delusion, whereas to me it was something very real and spiritually meaningful. How was I going to make sense of it all: delusion or reality? I spoke with local clergy, and even talked with my Bishop, hoping that he could throw some light on my experience, but they all saw it as a medical, rather than a spiritual, problem. If I spoke about my spiritual concerns to my doctors, this was seen as further evidence of psycho-pathology. I was living in a sort of no-man's-land without any spiritual help and I had two admissions to hospital under section because of major psychotic episodes, which led to my dismissal from my teaching post.

However, as a result of finding an antipsychotic medication which suited me, my condition finally stabilised about fifteen years after the trauma began. I was then able to return to teaching; and shortly afterwards I was finally told that, actually, I suffered from bipolar disorder, formerly known as manic depression (the same diagnosis as my brother's), although I also learned that for many years my hospital notes had recorded that I was suffering from schizophrenia!

In retirement I felt I needed to clarify, in my own mind, what the truth was about my experiences in 1973 and thereafter. By this time there was a wealth of literature available which looked into the matter of spirituality in a mental health context. The more I read, the clearer it became to me that my experience in church in 1973 had been a 'spiritual emergency': a term used to indicate an experience of sudden awareness of something deeply spiritually meaningful but which is completely overwhelming. The term only entered the mental health diagnostic manuals in the 1990s, about twenty years too late for me to be able to benefit from such a diagnosis. Unfortunately the observed symptoms presented by someone experiencing a spiritual emergency are very like those of someone having a psychotic episode, so a differential diagnosis can be difficult, even though very necessary to establish the most beneficial treatment plan.

It is encouraging to know that, in my local Trust now, a holistic approach to mental health care is in place. If necessary, my spiritual needs can be addressed by the Chaplaincy Team, alongside the medical care provided by a psychiatrist and his team of doctors and nurses. Some trusts have made provision for this for a long time now, and the need for such holistic care is recognised by the Royal College of Psychiatrists through its Special Interest Group in Spirituality. It is helpful to me to know that any spiritual support I might need will be provided by the Trust and will no longer, automatically and erroneously, be seen as an indication of a pathological condition.

It seems to me now that, because of my inherent genetic susceptibility to bipolar disorder, in 1973 I was on the verge of a manic episode as a defence against the stress, anxiety and low mood I was feeling (my psychiatrist's case notes at the time show that this was something he considered). I was certainly in a vulnerable state and this left me open to the spiritual dimension in a way that can be described as a spiritual crisis (or 'spiritual emergency', as now defined in the diagnostic guidelines).

This experience in 1973 changed my life; my wife attests to that. Some of the changes were destructive and painful for me and the whole family, but there has been much that has been positive and healing for us all. I realise that I am on a journey; looking back it is clear, now, that I was on a journey prior to 1973, without being aware of it, but suddenly, in a dramatic and traumatic experience, I was given some pointers to a meaningful way ahead.

To remain more or less symptom-free I have to take regular antipsychotic and antidepressant medication but live a fairly full life, enjoying the journey, caring for my wife – my wife for sixty years – who is now disabled with MS. Together we look forward to what lies ahead – here or beyond.

David Norman

OCD: Faulty formulas

OCD has no silver linings: it makes me neither house-proud nor tidy, careful nor precise. Rather, it makes me fearful, irritable, absent-whilst-present, unfriendly, antisocial.

There are no helpful quirks to a mental illness.

OCD is like an algebraic formula which stretches beyond the edges of my tiny brain: if X equals 3 and Y equals a heinous crime: how do I get myself out of this black hole?

Every few minutes, a new logic problem presents itself, demanding to be solved, sorted and filed away until the next time. Conversations with friends, auspicious moments, special looks: none of them are important compared to the desperate urgency of solving the latest vile riddle.

But how is my tiny brain to untangle the answer? Armed with half an equation, and missing some crucial variables, I set about to solve it. But how many mathematicians can claim to get it right first time? And isn't a hypothesis only proven by testing and trialling? So if I get one thought which worries me and another three which imply normality, surely it would be prudent to check again, reaffirm the conclusion…?

I've hit a snag in the procedure though: the more I recall, testing the variables, exchanging and disentangling the propositions, the more blurry they all become. X, Y and the rest of the sorry alphabet become more and more muddled until they're all arms and legs, and my own arms and legs are sore and weak from being held at strange angles during many long moments of 'checking'. We carry on this vicious little dance until, panting and fragile, I emerge from the tangle of thoughts, my breaths short and my hope severely stunted.

Who has won this round? In almost every case, this is an entirely needless question. It is always the victor.

How can I win at a game designed to floor me every time?

Thea Joshi

In the waiting

I am lying on the floor
fists pounding
into the ground
kicking and screaming
a fully-grown-adult tantrum –
wondering when you will hear me
wondering why I hear no response
why I hold my husband at arm's length
and entertain thoughts which dissolve into eternity around me.

Baulking at every person who assures me
God is not silent
but refuses to sit in the desolation of a crackly phone line.
Wondering why, when I am made in your image,
I am hounded by thoughts which split my head into a thousand pieces,
shards of who I was or who I could be
littering a wasteland.

Waiting for the tenderness of the One
who perceives the full, helpless state –
    and does not pull back –
waiting to be airlifted out of this infernal darkness
into eternal light.

Thea Joshi

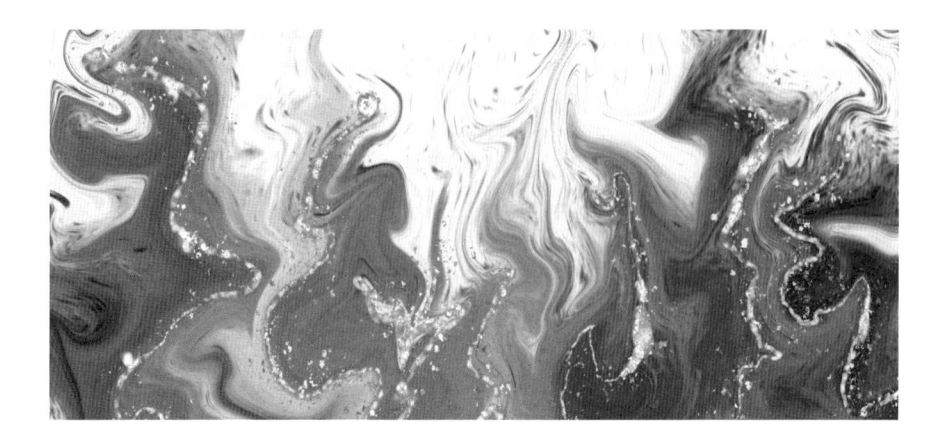

Anxiety

You said you knew what anxiety is?

You said you were nervous before your driving test.

You said you had butterflies in your stomach as you went on your first date.

You said you couldn't sleep the night before your maths exam.

But, my friend, that is not anxiety. That is just being nervous about a future event.

Let me tell you about anxiety:

Anxiety is crippling and devastating.

Anxiety is thinking the pavement will collapse under your feet and you will fall down into unmapped old mine workings.

Anxiety is standing on the beach and dreading the next big wave, as you are sure it will surge over where you are standing and wash you and your family away into the ocean.

Anxiety is not going into a shop because all the people in there will never be able to escape when a fire breaks out and you will be burnt alive.

Anxiety is avoiding elevators because the cables are sure to snap and the cabin will crash down the lift shaft until you experience the sudden jolt of death.

You laugh?

Yes, I know it is fantastic and improbable. But this is what I fear every moment of every day. It is an overwhelming feeling that chills to the core.

Part of me knows it is irrational – that it just doesn't make sense, but that part of me is drowned out by the paralysing terror that refuses to release me from its vice-like grip.

So that is why I take the pills.

John Butterfield, based on a conversation with a close friend

My purple monster

'Sometimes I wrestle with my monsters; sometimes we just snuggle.'
Anon

Monsters are only monstrous when they are hiding under the bed. Trust me, I know, I have one. My monster is a purple monster. It is sneaky. It is a small, coiled creature, nestled deep down in my subconscious. It is often hidden, but certain noises and tastes and overwhelming situations tickle my monster, irritating it until it erupts, until meltdown. My monster expands to fill all of the unoccupied space in my brain, its fur standing on end. It is a frightened cat, ready to pounce; a bird startled out of its nest; a dog growling and barking and snapping at an unexpected intrusion.

Let me explain. I don't really have a purple monster living in my head. But I am autistic[1], and I live with CPTSD[2], generalised anxiety[3] and situational depression.[4] Autism is a neurotype – a way of thinking and being. It is a diagnosis, but not necessarily a problem. Similarly, a counsellor recently helped me to understand my mental health labels not as disorders, but as rational responses to really painful and complicated situations. God made me autistic, and God celebrates my neurodiversity. The problem, for me, is that many people do not see mental health – or neurodiversity – that way.

That purple monster that I mentioned could be described as 'meltdowns'. For me, meltdowns are a part of autism. They will not be cured; I will not grow out of them. Autism can include differences in executive functioning, sensory experience, psychological processing and social interaction. For me, this includes finding it very tricky to organise my time; having no visual memory or sense of direction; needing to/being able to do multiple things at once; being able to make connections between seemingly unrelated facts (useful when you are doing a PhD!); hearing repetitive noises as louder than they actually are; relying on lip-reading and visual languages; being unable to stomach certain tastes and textures; having extreme empathy; and experiencing variable levels of social anxiety.

All of these things are part of who I am, and I don't dislike these parts of me at all. Many of these parts of me are gifts, or at least include a silver lining! But when society is structured around people who think and experience and live in a neurotypical way, those of us who are neurodiverse struggle. This world can be incredibly overwhelming. And, for me, that leads to the purple monster, to meltdowns, to a complete inability to cope, for a little while. Let me tell you about a few situations where my purple monster came out to play.

When I was nine, I called my teacher 'Mrs Thingamabob'. She was furious. I was sent out. I wasn't upset about being sent out. I was upset that I had upset her! She had written her name on the blackboard a few days earlier, so I was meant to remember it. I didn't. To me, this was the end of the world. If only Mrs Thingamabob had known that I have no visual memory, and that I cared deeply about how she felt, the purple monster would not have made me cry.

When I was twelve, my teacher told my mum that I never paid attention. Why? Because I refused to look at the board when he was teaching. Duh – I was listening! If I looked at the board, I got super confused, and had no idea what he was talking about. If I just closed my eyes and concentrated, though, my brain lit up with facts and connections that were light years beyond primary-seven grammar. If only Mr B had known that I loved learning and was perhaps focusing more than anyone else in that room, the purple monster would not have had a tantrum at my mum.

When I was eighteen, at music college, I had an argument with one of my teachers. She told me that I had to memorise the pieces that I was going to perform. I tried to explain that I couldn't. She said that that was nonsense, that everyone can memorise. I can't. If only I had known, back then, that I was autistic, and that reasonable adjustments were possible, the purple monster would not have made me storm out of my lesson.

When I was twenty-four, the educational psychologist who diagnosed my neurodiversity said that I should apply for Personal Independence Payment (PIP). I did. In the face-to-face interview, I performed 'well', talking with confidence and flair about my studies, my work and my hobbies. I also told the assessor that I couldn't drive without my wife in the car and that I needed adjustments around the house for my sensory and cognitive difficulties, amongst other things. Did I get PIP? Of course I didn't. If only the U.K. benefits system understood autism. If only the assessor knew that people with autism who were raised as female – which I was, though I now identify as transmasculine – mask our symptoms (we learn to hide our differences in order to fit into a patriarchal, normative world), the purple monster would be a little more manageable today.

The point is, I hide my purple monster because I have learnt to. I have been taught, throughout my life, that this world cannot cope with my differences, that I need to mask my monster if I want to succeed. Many people who are neurodiverse and/or experience mental health difficulties hide the ways in which we struggle to fit into, or to cope with, the inflexible ways of the places where we study, work and live. I will always be autistic, and experience the effects of CPTSD, anxiety and depression. But perhaps if I could hold hands with my purple monster as I went about my day, life would be very different. Perhaps if Mrs Thingamabob had taken the time to get to know me before assuming my ignorance, I wouldn't have had to worry so much about upsetting her. Perhaps if Mr B had been taught to attend to different learning styles, I would have been a better student. Perhaps if the classical music world actually talked about the vast amount of gifted musicians who are neurodiverse, the oppressive norms that it perpetuates could be dismantled. Perhaps if the systems that are supposed to support people with autism allowed me to afford assistive technology and reasonable adjustments, everyday stuff would be just that little bit easier and my wife might not have to be my carer, on top of working more than full time. Perhaps if autism were just that little bit more visible in this world, I could snuggle with my monster, instead of wrestling it.

As a minister, I often hear Christians say that they include everyone because 'We are all human'. They have a point. We are all human. But we are also all different. Perhaps if those differences were brought into the light, more people would feel genuinely included, actually welcome, fully represented, really alive. When Jesus healed lepers, he sent them to the temple to present themselves, to be seen. It's time for neurodiverse people to be presented to society, to be seen, to be accepted, to be included, to be loved, just as we are. We don't need to be healed. We need society to reconcile itself to our presence. Are you ready to be part of that change?

Action:

If you would like to help, here are some practical steps you could take. Several of these things are directly related to each of the experiences that I describe in this reflection:

1. Visit https://actuallyautistic.home.blog to learn more about autism.

2. Encourage those who work in education to learn about neurodiversity.

3. Point out gifts that often go unnoticed. For example, if you enjoy classical music, consider pointing out the emotive expression of the performer, or their funky purple shoes, rather than focussing on whether or not they have memorised their piece.

4. Offer affirmation, rather than criticism, to the neurodiverse people in your life.

5. Write to your MP about the discrepancies in the benefits system. Highlight the importance of taking neurodiversity and mental health seriously.

6. If you are a part of a church, consider taking steps to include neurodiverse people. For some ideas visit:
https://churspaciouscom.wordpress.com

Alex Clare-Young

Notes:

1. I was diagnosed with autism as an adult and identify as autistic and/or neurodiverse. Person-first language, such as 'Alex has autism', implies that autism is inherently problematic. Rather, I prefer to think of autism as a way of being which, for me, has both positive and problematic elements. The latter are intensified by a world which is structured around the needs and desires of neurotypical people – people who are not autistic.

2. CPTSD refers to complex post-traumatic stress. It is a presentation of PTSD in response to complex, repeating, or chronic micro-aggressions and/or trauma.

3. Generalised anxiety is a presentation of anxiety that is triggered by a range of stimuli or occurs without any trigger.

4. Situational depression is a presentation of depression that is triggered by particular situations.

Wounded healers

The rainbow man

I met the rainbow man when I was working in a night shelter for homeless men. The rainbow man dressed in bright colours – tie-dyed T-shirts, purple hair, pink nail polish. Spoke in colours. It was a depressing, colourless place – dingy, dirty yellow walls; clouds of grey cigarette smoke hanging.

He was labelled mentally ill, schizophrenic. At one time he had studied fine arts at college, somebody said, had worked masterfully in oils and acrylics. Now, he worked in Crayola crayon. Drew like a child: dogs and cats and upside-down pink-orange flowers planted in clouds. He got beat up by the men a lot.

One day he brought a leaf in from a walk he took (he was always taking long walks) and held it up to me and said to look, *see* the light in the leaf pulsing, dancing still.

I was busy and tired and had forgotten how to see, and said: 'Yeah, it's a maple leaf, so what' – there was someone buzzing at the door again, paperwork, so many important things to do. 'The light in the leaf,' he said again and danced away in a whirl of wind.

And when I sat down and stopped, I realised that what he meant was: to look and see that energy, that essence, alive in the leaf. He could see it. He was supposed to be disabled but he was able to see the light of God in a leaf and to wonder at it. After weeks of running blind through my life, the rainbow man taught me to open my eyes and heart again.

Neil Paynter

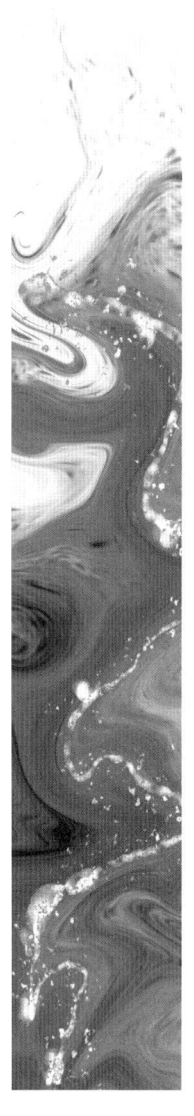

Elizabeth

I met Elizabeth while working in a psychiatric hospital. It was a place where few people kept track of the days. Either they were unable to – lost in a fog of heavy drugs – or, because the days were all the same, they didn't bother.

Elizabeth had an amazing and inexhaustible wardrobe and made a point of dressing up extravagantly. She sometimes changed as often as four times a day! And standing, smiling, in a long, flowing, golden gown, a floppy hat – both too big for the short old woman who looked like a little girl trying on her mother's outfits – long, white gloves, bright-red lipstick, costume pearls, dangling earrings in the shapes of moons and fishes, she explained proudly: 'I dress this way, darling, because the days are all the same. And if the dirty old days won't change then, by Jesus, I will!'

Through the long afternoons she danced. In the dirty, fold-up dining room. To a music only she could hear. All around her gathered the ghosts of the place: the suicides, the walking dead.

I danced with her sometimes when I was on duty and she taught me new steps. Taught me how to open up and hear the music. Taught me how to dance no matter what.

Neil Paynter

Maggie

'Maggie, you've got your teeth!'

Maggie stands in the fluorescent light of the homeless shelter and smiles, modeling them for us. 'Madonna, eat your heart out,' she says, and laughs in her husky, earthy way.

It's quite a contrast: the false perfection of the new, white-white teeth against the brown, wrinkled background of her crooked, beaten face.

It only took a year. 'Wait for your cheque.' 'Wait for your teeth.'

Maggie has learned patience. (Like everybody here, she's had to.) She knows it takes a long, long time for anything to trickle down to a night shelter in a basement. Having no teeth is a trial, but after so many trials and losses – abusive men, dead-end jobs, poor housing, psychiatrists and social workers, breast cancer; a best friend who lost all hope; a good friend who was murdered – you learn to endure, and to live with little things like having no teeth.

'You really look great, Mags,' I say.

'Well, thank you, dear, but they're just a plug in a leak, you know. The body dies, the soul is eternal, as they say. But at least I can chew now – no more soup and mush,' she says, and smiles brightly again.

'Alleluia,' I answer, and stop and gaze at her … But it's not her new white-white teeth I'm struck by – although I'm very happy she finally has them – it's her old laughing eyes – and the light that has never left her. The beautiful, strong light that no one has been able to blacken, or rob, or put out, or take away. The miraculous, amazing light she has, somehow, never lost faith in.

Neil Paynter

George

I met George when I was going to college and working part-time at a shelter for homeless men. When I wasn't busy, and he was free, we'd sit and talk together, about art and classical music. As a young man, George had studied oil painting. He'd wanted to learn to draw like the old masters, he told me. He loved the art of portraiture especially, and had dreamed of, just once, capturing a face so that it 'mirrored the soul'.

At first it seemed a little surprising to be talking about art and music in the cacophony of a night shelter, surrounded by bare, nicotine-yellow walls and ugly, orange linoleum scarred with cigarette burns.

I'd heard that George had been a soldier, too, that he'd fought at Normandy and in the Desert campaign, later again in Korea, but when I asked him about that period of his life, he said he didn't like to talk about it.

Once when Tommy was having a seizure, and lay writhing on the cold floor like he'd been shot, I glanced up and saw George. He gazed down at

Tommy and kept shaking his head; it was like he was away some place else. His face expressed infinite pity.

Blood drooled from the corner of Tommy's mouth; his body kept flailing and churning. 'Gonna be alright, Tom,' said George. Tommy roiled and writhed, his boyish, trenched face contorted, tortured-looking. George handed me his suit jacket, balled-up for underneath Tommy's head.

I tried to keep Tommy over on his side between attacks; with a tender, sore, caressing voice, George told Tommy that he was going to be all right, that he was just going to see the nurses.

'Just goin' to see the nurses,' the crowd of tough, scared men started up in a chorus. 'Tommy's just going to see the nurses.' 'Luck-y.' 'Some nice ones there, I'll bet ya.' 'Oh yeah, for sure.' 'Be alright now, Tommy.' 'Tommy, be alright.'

And, finally, the ambulance screamed up with a stretcher the paramedics rolled Tommy on to like a bag of loose sticks.

My colleague Phil, who'd been working on the front line for years, and knew George better than anyone probably, said that George felt profound guilt for having survived the wars – that George couldn't understand why he'd lived when all his good friends, and so many other good people, had been blown away or left crippled for life, had been taken prisoner and tortured, had gone missing and never been found ... He carried the question like a cross, Phil said.

'You see him alone sometimes, talking to himself, talking to God. Shouting at the heavens; praying for peace.'

A tabloid newspaper portrayed George as a dirty old drunk, on its front page one day. Some photojournalist shot him as he sat alone out on the front stoop of the shelter with a 'dead soldier' beside him. He looked like a poor, pathetic soul: dressed in a crumpled tweed jacket, bowed down by drink. The angle and light didn't do him justice, made his face look ugly and guttered. 'A Skid Row Alcoholic' the title underneath the picture read. There was a story concerning the growing number of homeless and the face of downtown. There was no report of him talking gently, humanly to Tommy as he lay writhing in hell, of the wars of liberation and absurdity he'd fought in through deserts and jungles and back streets; no mention that he had a wife and grown children somewhere, or of his dreams to become a fine artist who mirrored the soul.

No quote from him speaking knowledgeably, sensitively, passionately about the rich, beautiful, soaring music of Gustav Mahler.

The guys were mad. Somebody wanted to go down and teach the reporter a lesson. 'Give the poser a slashin'.'

Phil said it didn't surprise him. 'People have been painting him like that for ages now. Still hurt him though, I bet.'

George had one of the most beautiful faces I've ever seen. Sitting across from him one night, I told him that; I'd felt overwhelmed. He said thank you, that I was a gentleman.

It was hard to express with words. George's face was like grainy, grey rock, its features sculpted and etched by wind and rain, pocked and scarred by ice and snow; like an ancient landscape that had experienced fecund, young times of flowers; sudden rifts; slow, glacial change. George's face shone with the experience and wisdom of ages –

'Maybe that's what they mean,' said Phil. 'About suddenly seeing the face of Christ.'

Neil Paynter

Garry

A story from before digital cameras ...

'People ask me how I can always be so happy,' says Garry, and tells me his story.

About how some junkies broke into his basement room and stole his TV and music system. Stabbed him in the head and ribs sixteen times.

'I thought I was falling asleep, but I was really dying.'

'During it I had this feeling,' he says. 'Like someone suddenly reached out and touched me. My guardian angel, my mum said. And I knew I was safe and held in love.'

Sunlight falls on Garry's face and he closes his eyes; he says the stabbing helped to clear away the fog. 'People ask me how I can always be so happy – I'm back from death.'

He looks like he's on permanent vacation – standing in flowery knee-length shorts, leather sandals, and a T-shirt proclaiming LIFE'S A BEACH; a great smile across his broad tanned face.

We're standing in the middle of the city sidewalk. People run to important meetings; wait with clouded looks. Garry's bopping and dancing away …

I remind him about the last time I saw him. Down at the drop-in – pale and shivering in a corner, hugging himself.

'Ya, I wasn't a pretty picture, eh?'

Garry tells me he's moved on and hardly ever goes there now. He likes to go on long walks – round the park, the market, the botanical gardens … He's got energy to burn – energy he never knew he had.

'Here, look,' he says, and shows me the camera his father sent him for his birthday, turns it over in his knuckly hands like treasure. He laughs: 'I used to hate people taking my picture. I used to think I was ugly. Ugly from the inside out, you know? Now I wear my shorts, take my shirt off. Why not?' he says, and opens the zoom lens, 'there's nothin' to be ashamed of.'

Garry doesn't care if people see his scars, or think he's crazy or stupid.

'God thinks I'm beautiful. Jesus calls me his beloved son,' he says, like he has stood in front of God's gaze and grown bright with it. Like something brilliant has happened, and he'll never feel ashamed again.

I ask him what he likes to take photos of, and he says people he loves, things he loves: 'Sunsets and sunrises. Squares and fountains. Faces and flowers … I used to sit and watch TV. Now I wanna take pictures.'

Garry says he loves the way the light changes – and is everywhere. 'There's so much I never even noticed before. You know? … So, that's why I listen to jazz,' he says, and excitedly shows me his Walkman now. 'I used to listen to basement music – Black Sabbath, Iron Maiden. Now I listen to jazz. Walk around everyplace and take pictures and listen to jazz … I used to hate it. I didn't understand. The joy. The joy, but sadness too. Jazz people went through a lot, suffered. But it's the joy that comes through stronger in the end – Louis Armstrong, Ella Fitzgerald. I listen to the words. I never did before. They sink in. I used to hate it. I used to hate everything ... Life was a bitch. I didn't understand.'

Garry shrugs. 'Sometimes you gotta die to be born,' he says, and starts showing me the stack of photos he keeps in his backpack with a bottle of water; drops one the wind catches and carries off. 'Oh well, someone'll find it,' he laughs, as it Spirits away.

Garry says he was dead. Dead when they climbed in his casket and stole his buried treasure. Now his treasure is the light that glitters. Each new day. 'I just thank God ... See, listen,' he says, and reaches up and lays his hands on me: gives me his headphones.

'Can you hear? ...... See – light and dark. Sorrow and joy ... Can you hear?' he trumpets. People passing glance round, wondering if he's talking to them.

I listen. And can hear: the bluesy key, the brassy joy.

While I'm listening to the music of life, Garry stands out on the street corner handing out his photographs: waxy, shiny leaves of grass breaking up through concrete; blazing heads of flowers in a litter-strewn wasteland; the sun slowly rising up over office towers and apartment blocks ... Gives one to a woman who stops, taken aback ... then smiles as something slowly sinks in. Hands one to a man who lights up and laughs. He seems to know who to give them to: people stopped or slowed with care or worry; folk in a hurry who only have time for a bite. He seems to know: who needs energy, who needs some hope.

I close my eyes – and can see pictures in the music ...

I hand him back his halo.

Garry says when he walks through the mean street valley now he feels protected; he smiles, the lines and wrinkles around his eyes all crinkly and radiating out.

He looks lit up from within – his face beaming, his Hawaiian shorts like stained glass glowing.

The sun's out and the world is full of light. It seems to me that Garry is making it that way – and he is. We shake hands and he strolls off, listening to the sea of life.

I watch him disappear down the street, taking pictures of everything in the world he nearly lost.

Heading uptown everything is lit up from within. The crucified, leafy trees; the lined faces of souls ... Like a saint has passed this way trailing and spreading light. Like the fog has cleared.

There's a smell of tar; dazzle and glitter of sand dunes on a building site.

There's a gentle breeze and a warm, embracing feeling – I can feel the sun, sinking into my bones and heart. I want to run home and put my shorts on!

So why are you so happy? people passing seem to ask. I'm back from death ...

Neil Paynter

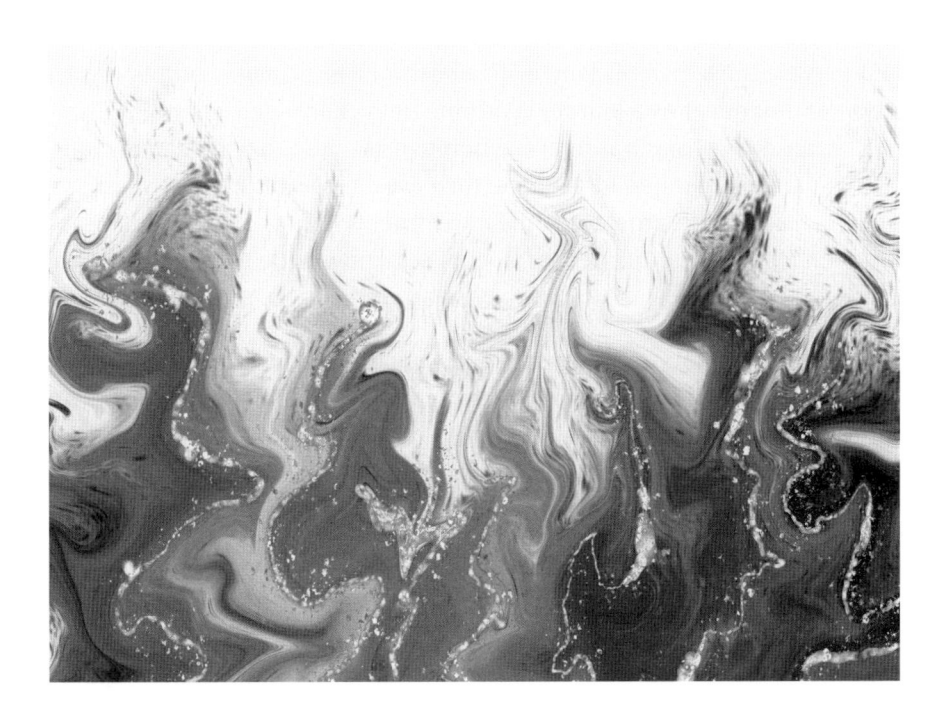

The Bible

Blessed are the poor in spirit

Depressive disorder is one of the most prevalent illnesses on the planet. According to the World Health Organisation, it is the leading worldwide cause of disability, affecting 300 million people; that is about 4 per cent of the world population.

Depressive disorder is not solely about feeling sad. Everyone feels sad sometimes, but depressive disorder also includes other aspects, including low motivation, low self-esteem, an inability to take pleasure or enjoyment in life, and feeling tearful, guilt-ridden and helpless. It can develop in response to difficult life events, or can happen for no apparent reason, when the delicate balance of mood which the brain normally maintains, becomes disturbed. For sufferers, life can become a dreadful, endless and hopeless treadmill.

So why would Jesus claim that such people, the 'poor in spirit', are truly blessed?

Obviously there are no simple pat answers to that question, but here is one thought on the subject. Many of those who have experienced depressive disorder describe it as a journey. With the help of anti-depressant medication, counselling, psychotherapy, cognitive therapy, personal reflection, patients are encouraged to examine their lives, their attitudes, their vulnerabilities, and to emerge from their treatment with a greater degree of emotional honesty and a deeper level of self-knowledge than was the case before.

As ever with mental health, there are no quick fixes, no easy answers; such exploration will not flick the switch and destroy the depression in an instant. Self-knowledge is for all of us a life-long quest. However, it is in these deepest regions of our minds and souls that God resides; radical self-knowledge surely therefore leads us to the purest form of prayer.

For this reason, the poor in spirit are on the brink of the Kingdom.

Gill Dascombe

Ezekiel

The prophet Ezekiel must have been a very colourful character. From the beginning of his book, he records strange and astonishing experiences. His call from God took place in the midst of a stormy wind. There was a cloud which contained a flashing light. He then had a vision of four living creatures, each with four faces, and wings with which they flew within a crystal dome. Later, he heard the voice of the Almighty, which, he says, was like the sound of many waters.

Many of his prophecies were accompanied by unusual, flamboyant actions, such as when he cut off all his hair, some of which he burnt, some he cut with a sword, some he scattered in the wind and some he sewed into the hem of his robe.

Ezekiel's experiences and character have led some to speculate that he may have had a psychotic illness, perhaps bipolar disorder. However his eccentric behaviour was not out of place in his time and culture. Indeed, the Hebrew word to prophesy can also, in some translations, mean to rave, or to act like a 'madman'.

Ezekiel's message to Israel, however, was an important one which was full of hope and optimism. He was adamant that, despite her disobedience, trauma and exile, she was not condemned to eventual destruction, but to new life, and a new heart, a message as incredible and wonderful as the vision of the valley of dry bones coming to life which inspired it.

W.F. Albright, the Old Testament scholar, wrote this about Ezekiel:

> 'He was one of the greatest spiritual figures of all time, in spite of his tendency to psychic abnormality – a tendency which he shares with many other spiritual leaders ... A certain "abnormality" is required to divert ... thoughts and ... emotional experiences from the common treadmill of human thinking and feeling.'[1]

Gill Dascombe

Note:

1. *From the Stone Age to Christianity: Monotheism and the Historical Process*, William Foxwell Albright, The Johns Hopkins University Press, 1957

Consider the lilies of the field

All of us, whoever we are, experience anxiety. It is a common, natural emotion, arising in the deepest parts of the brain, as part of our instinctive response to danger or threat. The familiar physical symptoms of a racing heart and churning stomach represent the body's preparation for fight or flight.

A certain amount of anxiety is healthy; it boosts our performance in response to the demands and responsibilities of life. But for some of us, some of the time, that healthy mechanism can run out of control and begin to dominate everything. We constantly anticipate the worst, constructing endless scenarios to combat the unknown, but end up not protected, but controlled, by endless, ceaseless, unbearable, imprisoning worry.

So what are we to do?

'Can any of us by worrying add a single hour to life?' asks Jesus. Actually, just the opposite. Medical opinion tells us that excessive anxiety can lead on to physical illness: heart disease, diabetes or cancer, for example.

And while we are worrying about the future, we are not experiencing the present. Because a life spent in anxiety will not have been lived: it will have been avoided; we will never be fully present to any experience, but always exist in a threatening and illusory future. A life spent in anxiety will be spent in the dark shadows of imagination, not in the clear light of reality.

Jesus' words about anxiety often get misconstrued, and end up doing no more than making people feel guilty for not being able to 'pull themselves together'. I don't believe that Jesus wanted that. But I do believe he wants us to take responsibility for our lives, including our emotional lives. This is not easy. Managing our worries and fears is a long haul, a lifetime's work, and we should never be afraid to seek the help of others.

The key, however, is very simple. It is all around us. The key is learning to accept ourselves as we are, and to value and live in the reality of the present moment.

Like the sparrows of the air and the lilies of the field.

Gill Dascombe

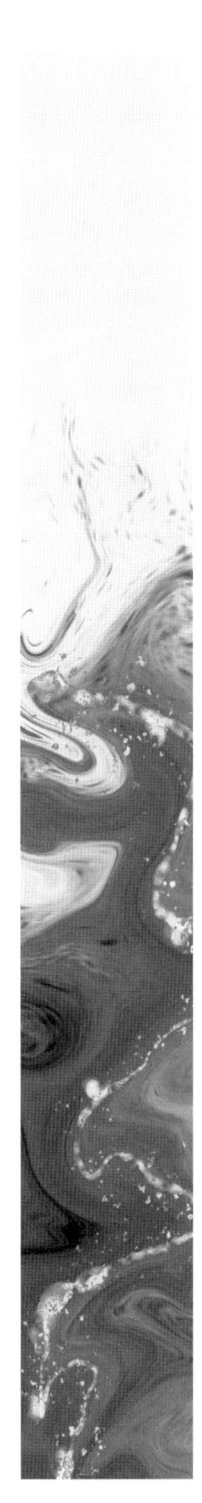

The Gerasene schizophrenic

It seems possible, from the description of his symptoms, that the man whom Jesus met wandering amongst the tombs in Gerasa (Mark 5:1–20) may have been suffering from schizophrenia. He exhibits a characteristic paranoia (suspicion of others) and severe anxiety. His famous description of being not one person but a 'legion' may refer to the constant torment of hallucinatory voices, from which he appears to have sought relief by his restless wandering and apparent self-harming. This harrowing existence is akin to a kind of living death, rather like living in a graveyard amongst the tombs.

He had been shunned by his home village, abandoned by his community and left alone to wander in a lonely and spiritless place. Even today, in our so-called rational and scientific age, people who have severe and enduring mental illness often find themselves excluded and marginalised by society. Typically, they fall rapidly down the socio-economic scale; at the mercy of a complicated and uncompassionate benefits system, they frequently inhabit the poorest housing and are consigned to live in the most deprived areas.

The sad truth is that, then as now, many people are scared of mental illness and choose to turn their back on those who are affected, thereby adding to the burden of their distressing and trying symptoms, social isolation and stigma.

Jesus healed the man, driving out his demons, and the astonished villagers came upon him clothed and in his right mind.

But there is another aspect to this miracle, whose potential we see, but whose outcome is hidden. The terrified villagers drove Jesus back to his boat and begged him to leave them alone. Caught up in the hostility and chaos, the terrified man begged Jesus to take him along, as a disciple.

But Jesus refused. 'Go home to your friends' he said, 'and tell them how much the Lord has done for you.'

Friends? This angry mob? Would he have the courage?

And would they have the courage to overcome their fear, accept him back, and restore the schizophrenic to his place within their community as someone with much to contribute?

If they can, then the miracle will be truly complete!

Will they? Will we?

Gill Dascombe

The woman who was bent double (Luke 13:10–13)

I've often wondered about the story of the woman Jesus healed in that reading: Why was she bent over? What was the spirit that crippled her? I wrote a story for her 30 years ago. It was based on some of the women I met while I was working in homeless shelters and hostels, and in working on it for today I have brought into it some of the women I have met latterly as a therapist. I have learned so much from some of these women and I hope this story does them justice.

A man came up to her in the park and asked where mummy was,
'Over there feeding the ducks with Jimmy,' she said.
'Shall I show you where the baby ducks are?'
'Oh, yes please,' she said.
So he took her hand
She could still see mummy and Jimmy
And they went towards the bushes.

She didn't know what to do
She knew he shouldn't have done that
At first she just thought he looked silly
Until he touched her
She wanted to scream, but nothing came out
He told her it was a secret
and she must never tell

She wasn't sure about that,
but she didn't let mummy see the blood
in case she got into trouble.

She didn't notice then,
but she didn't really look ahead of her any more
She just kept her eyes on the ground
so no one could see her
And people said what a sweet little girl she was.

The priest at church
said he was short of people to serve on the altar
She'd watched the boys do it so many times
She wanted to do it for God
It took her a few weeks to pluck up the courage
and then she waited behind one Sunday
'I'd like to help,' she said.

Why hadn't he said you had to be a boy?
How could she have known?
He pretended to be kind,
but she'd seen that smile before.
She bowed her head.

It was in a geography lesson
she suddenly realised her seat was damp
She couldn't understand it
And then the awful horror flowed through her
and from her
She tried to sit there tidying her books
till everyone had left
But Mr Parsons kept Rawlings behind
and she couldn't stay any longer
So she ran
but Rawlings saw
And the boys pointed at her and laughed for months
and called her dirty
and she bent her head a little more

She started at 'the works' down the road
as a filing clerk
so proud of her first wage packet
Tony had just started in the office next door
After their second week he asked her out
She sat down and opened her wage packet while he got the drinks
He laughed when he saw her payslip
'Is that all you get?'
'Why, what do you get?'
It wasn't much but it was more than her
and she knew he did exactly the same work
Her head bowed a little more

She enjoyed the Christmas party
she was happy to stay and help clear up at the end
The man with ginger hair from purchase control stayed too
She didn't like him much
He offered to help her carry some of the chairs back to the canteen
She hadn't realised how drunk he was

She pushed him away and ran
He shouted after her
'If you tell anyone they'll never believe you
and new jobs aren't so easy to find nowadays'
She ran home, bent her head and cried.

She saw more of Tony
She managed to get transferred to another office
She got promotion, supervised a small team,
enjoyed work most of the time

Tony proposed
it seemed only natural to accept
She thought she'd like to keep her own name
but Tony was having none of that
– of course it was a silly idea really

The wedding day was a bit of a blur
but she did promise
– with her head bowed before God –

to obey him.
Tony reminded her of that
– Often.

He said it would be easier if they just had one bank account
so she might as well transfer all her money into his
Of course, she must bend to his wishes now.

He came home late one night, very drunk
She had been worried about him
He was angry
how dare she not trust him
He tipped the ashtray over her head
He knew she hated the smell of his cigarettes
She bent over and retched

Being pregnant made her feel worthwhile
She had thought she might work part-time after the baby was born
But Tony pointed out how stupid that was
and Mr Frazelli explained how impossible a job-share would be
She hadn't quite understood the explanation,
but still … she bowed to his superior knowledge

Tony drank a bit less after Bobby was born
he seemed quite happy for a while
then he lost his job
she was never quite sure why
She did ask but he punched her in the stomach
and told her it was none of her business
she doubled up and he hit her with a saucepan
which caught something in the middle of her spine
She found it hard to stand properly for very long after that

She didn't like him touching her any more
One night she tried saying 'no'
She didn't know how she was still alive in the morning
Bobby was toddling now and came to find her
hidden – bent – in the garden shed
He cried when he saw her

her silent tears bubbled slowly
she bent lower

But she knew she couldn't put Bobby through this any longer

She didn't go back into the house
She took Bobby's hand and went to the police station
'A domestic affair madam'
'Very difficult for us to intervene'
'Shouldn't have married him should you?'
'Can't be that bad surely'
'Cup of tea before you go?'
She bent lower – and left

Bobby was hungry and she had no money
– if only her mum was still alive …
She wasn't sure how to claim social security money
At the office she waited
and waited
A man offered her a can of super lager
but it seemed best to refuse
Eventually someone called her name and gave her a form to fill in
And she waited some more

'You haven't filled in your address on this form'
'I don't have one'
'We can't process this without an address
where would we send the money?'
She bent lower and got up to walk away
'Why don't you try Women's Aid?' he called after her

It took her a while to pluck up enough courage
to ask someone for 10p for the phone
'… Wed and Friday evenings,
if you would like to leave your name and number
we'll call you back as soon as possible …'
She let the phone drop and bent lower

She stood outside the church for a while
It wasn't the one she used to go to
She hadn't been for a long time

Tony liked a long lie on Sundays and she couldn't leave Bobby
She went round to the manse
'… you did promise …
… for the rest of your life …
… what God has joined …
… find it in your heart to forgive him …'
The phrases floated round her like a red mist
She stumbled out and bent lower

She sat in the church with Bobby
it was only open because the cleaner was in
so she wouldn't be able to stay long
at least it was dry
although not very warm
Perhaps she should pray
'Father God …'
No, she couldn't pray to a man
How could he possibly understand?
She bent her head to the ground and wept

Bobby had torn a page out of the Bible
That would mean more grief from someone
She looked at the page
she knew the story,
but she'd never really thought about it before
Here was a man who cared about
and respected women
it was a long time since she'd met one of those

She knew how that woman felt
bent double with grief and pain
unable to look anyone in the eye
but Jesus called her over
She imagined Jesus calling her by her name
What would that be like? –
in a place where only men were important
'I have called you by your name
you are mine'
that came from the Bible surely?

And Jesus reached out to the woman
with compassion and understanding
he cared about her
he had noticed her!
And he wasn't making fun of her
'You are set free,' he said
Imagine
freedom from fear
freedom from pain
freedom from shame
freedom to be herself
It hardly seemed possible.
To be free of her memories
to be free of Tony
to be free to teach Bobby a different way to be a man.

'Immediately she stood up straight,' it said
– what must that have been like?
Not only to stand straight for the first time in years
but to look into Jesus' eyes
to look into Jesus' eyes and see respect
to look into his eyes and know that she was seen
truly seen
known
and accepted.

The crowd had started to heckle Jesus
he wasn't playing by the rules
and what did he do?
He was angry, he called them 'hypocrites'
He told them that the woman's needs were more important
than their stupid rules.
Her needs mattered.
Imagine that
she mattered.
Could that really be true?
Jesus actually got angry
with the people who didn't think her needs mattered

Reflections and stories 153

And he called her 'a daughter of Abraham'
She wasn't sure what he meant by that
but it didn't sound quite right somehow

The cleaner was putting her coat on
She knew she'd have to leave
but where would she go?

'You look worn out hen
and the wee boy can't keep his eyes open
haven't you got a home to go to?'
She looked at the cleaner
and slowly shook her head
And the cleaner looked at her
right into her eyes
just as Jesus must have done when the woman straightened up

She knew
the cleaner knew
knew what had happened to her
'I'm only round the corner if you fancy a cup of tea'

The house was tiny
but it was warm
and safe
Bobby ate some bread and jam
and fell asleep
she didn't know how she'd ever get him moving again
when they had to leave

The cleaner saw the torn piece of paper
from the Bible in her hand
and took it from her
'That's a good story that one
– "daughter of Abraham" –
that's what he said

I like that
My granny told me he said it
because all the men were "sons of Abraham"

but that was a new one
"daughter of Abraham"
that was all Jesus' own idea
to include the women
and the men didn't like it at all.'
The cleaner smiled

'And he got angry
about them thinking their rules mattered
more than people
I like that
I reckon he'd be pretty angry about those bruises of yours
nobody deserves that'

'No,' she said, hesitantly
'No, nobody deserves that'
and she started to feel something strange and new.
This woman was right
'NO, NO, I DON'T DESERVE THAT'
she couldn't remember when she had last felt angry
she had been too tired
too bent
but now …

The wee cleaner was talking again
'I went into care when my granny died
– "care!" – there wasn't much of that there

When I left
I decided I might as well make money
doing what I'd had to do there for nothing
I didn't know much else
but it was rough on the streets
heroin helped block out what I was doing
made it easier
but then I needed more money to buy it
so I needed more punters
and more heroin.

I've been clean a good few years now
I met a woman who saw me
really saw me
I thought she was just one of those daft Christians
– well she was –
but she wasn't daft

She saw beneath the slap on my face
beneath the streetwise hooker
beneath the strung out addict
she saw me like my granny saw me
and maybe like Jesus saw that woman

You can stay here for a few days if you want
you and the wee one will have to sleep on the couch
there's no spare room
but it'll give you time to sort things out a bit'

She lifted her head and looked at the cleaner
and she knew
she had just met the Risen Christ
in a wee old cleaner
an ex-heroin addict
who'd sold her body on the streets

Here was the face of Christ
Here for her
Accepting her
Longing for her to be whole
Embracing her in her brokenness
And setting her free

She knew it would be a long road back
No – not back
Forwards
Forwards with Bobby
And with a new friend

Linda Hill

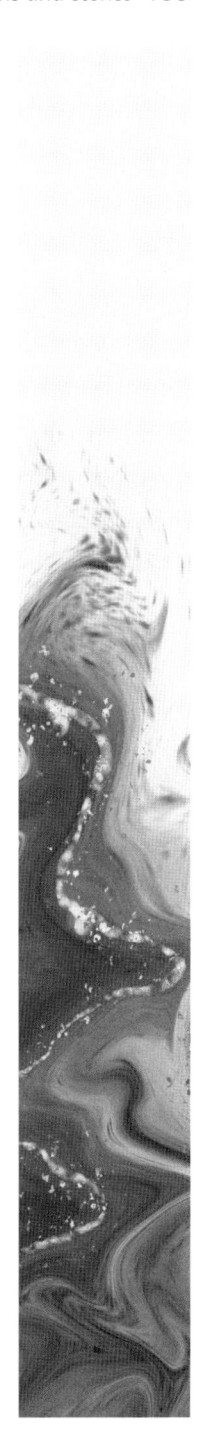

The aftermath of violence: Jephthah and his daughter

(Judges 11, 12:1–7, especially 11:30–40)

Introduction:

The imaginative interpretation of this difficult passage of scripture is based on the effects of living as a young person with a badly damaged survivor of the Second World War and subsequent trauma. We would now call this severe post-traumatic stress disorder (PTSD), and the effects it can have on the second and third generation is itself studied, as it has affected some societies.

Jephthah is seen here as the product of adverse childhood experience, and then the effects of militia life at a young age. His family of origin wanted him back only when he was useful to them, and seem to have taken no further responsibility for him, and neither did his society, both features experienced by ex-soldiers of formal and informal armies.

The inability to see beyond himself and his own perceived requirements is at the core, and a consequence is his immediate blame of the party who will suffer at his hands, in a reversal of parental duty. His particular understanding of God as brutal and unchangeable may have helped his survival in war but meant he was a poor interpreter of the affective nature of God, who asks for no sacrifice, and permits no one to sacrifice another in God's name. In war as in peacetime.

While many Old Testament stories show the effects of unhealed wounds down the generations, in this case the personal family suffering ends with the daughter, but the societal damage is remembered, even when her name is forgotten and her father recalled only as war leader and inauspicious peacetime official.

Suffering undealt with can cause harm down the generations.

Forgiveness does not heal. They are different. Forgiveness is born of will and of action; it may assist healing, but cannot replace it.

Many stories in scriptures speak of suffering down the generations where hurts are unresolved or evil deeds not acknowledged. With the stories of Abraham's sons, Ishmael and Isaac, we may feel anger at the failed parent. There is the trafficked child with no name in the house of the Syrian commander Naaman, who tells where he may gain healing, but whose name and tale are not told. The stories speak to us of damage done to the human psyche by war, by fleeing for safety when young, then or now, and how such traumas can entrap a person.

Jephthah's daughter:

This is my tale.

I am Jephthah's daughter. I have no name, no descendants. I had a mother, but her name is lost too.

My father's suffering did not endure the generations, for there were none. I do not know if the suffering of my cousins, and the other children of violence, ended with their lives. Or whether it is passed on.

I was a child of the Promised Land. My people had crossed the sea and desert, and survived. I knew the stories of old – of Abraham sending out his firstborn to die with his mother in the desert; of Abraham believing God called for his surviving child to be sacrificed – and finding himself wrong.

I came later, and was not so blessed. I am remembered, but as a symbol. I am to many the model of the passive, virtuous, obedient young girl, obedient to God and to my father. In this way I did not need a name. Others blame God for my death.

There is a balm in Gilead – but not for Jephthah of Gilead, nor his daughter. Nor for those who assail me again with this image of me, and of the violent deity of duty they have set up behind me.

Behind my tale lies the pain that made Jephthah what he became. The pain that limited his life, so his final years bore no fruit. Some pain only God can heal.

Jephthah, my father, was an Ishmaelite, born first and outside marriage. He was still young, his brain not fully formed, his body not yet at adult strength, when his father died and his half-brothers threw him out. He fled for his life, leaving behind his possessions, his inheritance, his friends.

He survived. 'God opens, God releases' is the meaning of his name. Did that happen? He gathered a band, taking in those on the edges, those deemed worthless. He became a warlord in the hills. He was good at this.

They were effective. What things did he see, what did he do in those years, that turned his mind hard? That gave him those headaches, the bad days when my mother hid me away?

Yet, my father settled, and had a home.

There were good days in that house too. But always with him at the centre. His mind had focused inwards, and he could not escape it. He could not see other lives, living beside him. For him we existed in how he saw us, in his mind. In that house, his mood was everything.

Then came the terror times, of war at hand. The family who rejected him, the family whose flocks he had harried, they needed a leader, and called for him. He knew war: he was their best chance.

He came, but negotiated. There were to be conditions. He would be their leader, at war, and afterwards their judge. He, the rejected, was now more powerful than they. He was no mercenary hired for cash, but a man with a stake in the nation.

They had no choice. They swore they would accept his terms, at the shrine, before God.

He was wiser than they. He negotiated. He sent envoys to the enemy. The envoys spoke of battles long past; and of what they led to: the boundaries and rights of safe passage, the borders agreed by compromise, and the route away from violence. He invoked the God of all to be the judge.

They did not seek peace. He negotiated with the god in his mind, asked victory, and offered a price. He routed his enemies from the rear. For that triumph, with the sense of God strong in him, he was at last revered among his brothers and their people. But he had made a vow to God. It was a vow that God did not ask for, did not wish, and was not Jephthah's to make.

The price he offered the god he bargained with was not his to give. He had sworn to sacrifice to his image of God the first living thing that crossed his path when he came back to the quiet safety of home.

No one has the right to swear like that. No parent has the right to destroy their child's life – by murder, neglect, or the pain that will limit their life forever. The young have the greater right, to life in its fullness. The Law says it is worse for a parent to kill their child than for a child to kill their parent.

I did not know of that oath, not then. High in the hills, we heard good news, of battles won and peace achieved. We learnt that we were safe again, and he would return.

So for his coming I thought to surprise him, placate him, welcome him. I was his pet, his only child, the delight of his eyes and his hope for grandsons. I wanted to show affection and warmth after his wars.

I surprised him. He saw me coming, rejoicing. Singing and running to embrace him.

I did not know of his idol, nor his blasphemy; nor that he saw only himself in the story, that war had broken his mind.

So when he saw my dancing, felt my embrace, he recoiled. Sorrow and shame were before him. In war you manage your shame by blaming those you slaughter, the women who get in the way, the children who can be expended, and chasing frightened boys to their deaths is collateral damage.

I had brought horror upon him. I was to blame. All he could see was himself. His survival, his honour, his view of God.

And now his last chance of descendants. His name would die. I was the cause of his misfortune. He blamed me for that.

Yet he wanted my comfort, my assent to what he had sworn.

He'd not asked me. But there was no way out. So, I did what I learnt from my father. I negotiated. Don't give me a year to marry a man of his choice and bear a child. I asked: Wait two months. No more.

I did not want to spend them in his house. I could not yet forgive him. I gave assent with my words as I have been taught, the dutiful daughter. I gave him my rejoicing – now I needed time for the rejoicing in my life and my time of grieving an untimely end.

'I am not the Ammonites who occupy your mind, waking and sleeping, whom you must kill to live yourself. I am real: I have a different life – which you will take from me. I will go to the high mountains, with those who care for me but have no say in the great plans of life. Then you can have your way, your violation of my right to live.

'Will my uncles come to save me? Will your kin, your brothers and their sons, keep their word to you? And will they cherish and support you, pray for your damaged mind after your damaged actions? Or will you be pariah among them when they feel they cannot cope? Will they run from you, avoid you? What deity is yours that would demand all this?'

His family had the duty and the chance to save my life, to save him from himself. They did not come. His warrior band, his wider people, had that chance. They did not act. The priests had the summer months to advise him, speak to him of the living God, help him to repent. They were silent. All failed me, and they failed him too. They used him as they needed him, but gave nothing back.

I met God in the hills. In those months borrowed from death I met the living, breathing source of kindness. God spoke to me, in the small things of life: the spring flowers in the grass, the birds in the bushes and the small creatures. God spoke in the big things: in the sunsets and stars, wind in the trees, and the two full moons. God does not limit life but increases it.

Though I was angry at first. I had done my duty to the savage god of barren oaths, who wrenched my youth from me, had taken all love, all respect for my father from me. I wanted to be away from my father and his god; among the girls who saw my side of the tale, who had fathers formed in those wars. I was angry at the darkness Jephthah had met in his life that had shrunk his mind and made his emotions turn inwards, to survival at all costs, to an image of a god who demands the impossible. I was angry for that grey hard centre of his mind, that could not listen to others where the heart was concerned, that had crippled life at home. When he was away at war I had longed for his return – but the house was lighter for his going. That lightness had made me joyous that final, fateful day.

In the hills I was not in his shadow – but as God created me. The last blasphemy is to slaughter the future. I was barren of the chance of children – but my life was not barren before God.

I could not change the practices of power, and my voice would not be heard. I could not change Jephthah in his absorption with his suffering. But I freed myself from that vision of God, and in that I found myself. They did not come to chase me to death: when the months were passed I met them to their faces, set my eyes to the hills of hope and spoke no more.

What happened next? God did not show pleasure. War did not end. The men of Ephraim came to Jephthah's house in their need and contempt. They said they would burn his house, his last place of safety, the place to grieve its silence, destroy his place of memories, if he would not fight again. So, with no hope left and no respect of men, he fought to ease his pain. There were no vows to any gods. In that civil war, he slaughtered our own people.

The bread of adversity lay in my lifeless body, barren of food for his soul. The wine of violence was poured out with my blood, bringing death.

Jephthah was then Judge in Israel. God's judge and leader of the people. Judgement scarred by his betrayal of parenthood, the sacred gift. Who trusted him in judgement? Who saw the Seat of Mercy behind his actions? Did he cling to an image of God which is not the kindness of God? Did he ask God for mercy, his daughter for forgiveness?

Jephthah judged Israel for six years. Then he died, with no Sabbath year of rest and relief, and went home to his fathers.

What of his brothers, who had used him, given him power? Did they feel remorse? Did the pain travel the generations?

What of those who followed me to the hills? The grieving of young girls continued, nameless like me in the chronicles of power, but they told of a story remembered among the voiceless, the illiterate, the ones who no one hears.

Later, a man named Jesus healed children, those with loving parents, or burdensome parents, or helpless parents; and others with no one to speak for them. For him, love grew in action, the balm of Gilead for all, the healing that allowed forgiveness to flow.

I am Jephthah's daughter, collateral damage of a war that damaged my father's mind and his knowledge of God. I have a name before God. I was expendable to men. Not to God.

Rosemary Power

Contending with God (Genesis 32:22–32)

As I seek to deal with the spiritual fallout of being a primary caregiver for our adopted son, I have come to appropriate this story of Jacob wrestling with God before crossing the River Jabbok to face a difficult challenge.

When Teddy was placed with us for adoption at the age of 18 months, we were told that he had some 'delays' that he would likely grow out of as he got older. However, these 'delays' proved to be major medical, emotional, mental issues that began to exhibit themselves at the age of seven.

Over the next few years, he was diagnosed with approximately 18 different conditions, including 'mental retardation', bipolar, explosive behaviour disorder, verbal apraxia, and Fetal Alcohol Syndrome (his birth mother apparently drank while pregnant, which resulted in brain damage to Teddy). As a result of this almost 'toxic' mix of conditions, Teddy has spent the majority of his life residing in some sort of psychiatric residential centre. And, if these conditions were not enough of a challenge for him (and for us), one month before his 18th birthday, he was diagnosed with Stage Four germ cell cancer, and endured two major surgeries and six months of intensive chemotherapy treatments.

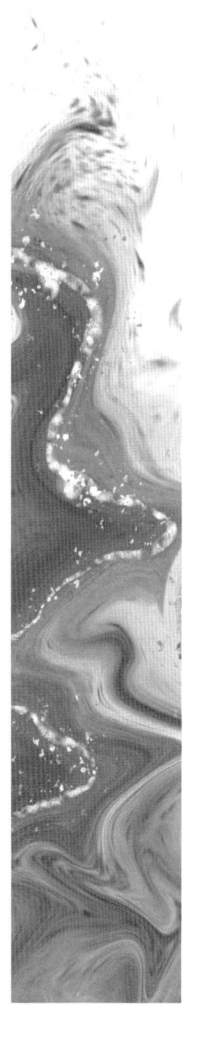

Despite the particular circumstances of our son's conditions, we share much in common with all caregivers. We went from a seemingly average family, to one dealing with profound crises. We have endured an emotional roller coaster, which seems to come to the end of the ride only to start climbing up the track almost immediately. Despite pretty good major medical coverage, we have incurred tremendous debt in seeking, finding and trying to provide resources for our son. And because of the fact that for roughly ten years we have had to travel two hours in each direction to visit Teddy in whatever facility he had been placed in, at least once a week, my wife and I have aged physically far more quickly than we might have expected.

Like many caregivers, the challenges of trying to care for a beloved member of our family also confronted the spiritual side of our lives. My wife and I are both strong Christians, and I am a Presbyterian Church (USA) pastor. Yet those 'credentials' did not exempt us from having to wrestle with how our faith responds to the difficulties with which our son struggles and how we could provide the best possible care for him. The particular circumstances of our son's conditions, and the almost immediate confrontations we had with the medical and educational communities in seeking help for him, did not allow us to go through the typical denial stage of caregiving. Yet it was interesting to see how some of the experts had trouble recognising that someone as young as seven could have profound mental and developmental issues. ER staff, psychiatric workers, teachers all seemed to want to pass off our son's conditions as simple tantrums (until they experienced his out-of-control violence personally).

It was also a fascinating experience to see how other people of faith responded to the situation. For some, there seemed to be the easy answer of prayer. While I strongly believe in prayer, I came to realise that God's answers came in the form of staff, facilities and programmes which could provide services. Our job became, in a sense, to get off our knees and get busy finding these resources.

We also encountered folks who were sure an exorcism would cure our son; as well as some legal folks who could not understand that mental illness was not going to be cured in someone like Teddy. It seemed others were more in denial than we were.

Thom M Shuman

Waiting and hope

Psalm 31:9–10, 24

When he was 17, our son, Teddy, was living in a residential facility for people with mental and developmental disabilities. I was planning on taking him out one Saturday morning, and when I called earlier in the week to arrange that, the staff informed me that he had a lump on the side of his neck. So, I arranged to take him to see our family physician on Saturday morning. The doctor, who was also a friend, examined Teddy and said he thought it was an enlarged gland and would refer us to a specialist.

About 12:30 that night, the doctor called me to say that he could not get to sleep – and wanted me to take Teddy down to the Children's Hospital for immediate examination the next morning. We did, and long story short, they kept him overnight; and the next morning, after further testing by several doctors, we were told that Teddy had Stage 4 germ cell cancer. And thus, we began a journey that no child and no parents should ever have to take.

Teddy endured two major surgeries and six months of intensive chemotherapy before the doctors felt that they had got all the cancer.

I remember sitting in the waiting room while he went through his first surgery.

It had been a whirlwind 24 hours from discovering what we thought was a minor issue was actually a life-threatening one; from talking with one doctor after another, until we sat around a table with all of them to hear that devastating diagnosis. And as I sat in that uncomfortable chair, flipping through magazines whose words and pictures I never noticed, I wondered 'How will we get through this?' And hope walked into the room in the guise of a friend, who simply came over and sat down next to us. And was with us until the operation was over.

I remember standing by the bed as Teddy was about to begin his first round of chemotherapy. What would it do to him? How would his body handle it? How could someone with limited cognitive abilities understand what was going on? Would hope be in that room, in that treatment? And then one of the oncologists came in, a young man who wore a yarmulke, and we just stood there in silence on either side of Teddy's bed. And then he simply reminded me that our common faith tradition called us to wait, in hope, for God. And then he left the room, leaving the gift of his hope in my heart.

I remember those sleepless nights spent in Teddy's room with him, watching the chemotherapy slowly drip into his body, listening to his soft breathing, hearing his occasional question, 'Am I going to die?' And I wondered if hope had simply abandoned him, and us. And then, a nurse would come in to check on him, take his vitals, and hold his hand, reassuring him that he was not alone, that he was surrounded by caring, compassionate hope.

I remember sitting in the family room on the oncology unit, taking a break from the fears, the worries, the hopelessness that threatened to seep into my heart and stay there. And a family would come in with sandwiches, snacks, or a home-cooked meal. Families who had been in this same place, in the same situation. They would share their stories, some of celebration and others of heartbreak. But as they left the room, I discovered that what they had really fed me was hope.

Long ago, this unnamed psalmist, going through a similar situation of struggling with heartache and loss, filled with questions and fears, overwhelmed by doubts and worries that left them lying awake at night, penned these simple words about trusting in God, and waiting … cradled in God's hope.

With shattered souls
and hearts hollowed by loneliness,
with knees numb from kneeling
at bedsides and empty chapels
and hands aching from holding tight
to others through the night,
with lips longing to sing
and minds empty of the words,
we wait, we wait, we wait
for you and the hope
you shape from your own
tears.

Thom M Shuman

Young people

A day in the life … Patrick: children and young people therapist

Patrick is a systemic therapist with a background in social work and child mental health with the NHS. Since he retired, he volunteers with Freedom from Torture's Children, Young People and Families team two days a week, holding face-to-face therapy sessions with children and adolescents.

A blog by Patrick, from the Freedom from Torture website:

At present I have 15 clients, children and young people who have sought sanctuary in this country. Some come in once a week, others maybe just once a month. That's a good sign, if someone feels that they have no need to see me each week.

Some come alone, others with family members. For those with families, I will have agreed with the parents how much I am going to focus on children and how much I am going to focus on the family.

Generally, there is an interpreter present, because most of our clients do not have English as a first language and can only speak of their experiences in their mother tongue.

In a typical day I will see four clients. I have to plan all the sessions beforehand and I have to be prepared for whatever may happen.

I have been using the Eye Movement Desensitisation and Reprocessing (EMDR) treatment method for Post-Traumatic Stress Disorder (PTSD), a therapy that I have used for several years.

An EMDR session is an hour and a half. But first I spend some time with the client catching up on how life has been treating them, as they are often marginalised socially and economically. Then we run the EMDR session.

I need to be prepared for anything that might come up. Finally, I have to have enough time to settle the client before they leave. Sometimes a client dissociates during the session. They don't know where they are or they think they are back with the torturer being tortured again. Some people do it temporarily. You see them go. A good interpreter sometimes can see it and alert you.

I will stop whatever is happening and actually bring them back to the room. I may end the session, putting it on hold so the client is able to leave and is able to manage until the next session.

We have quite a lot of support in the team. We have individual case management from the team manager. We have peer supervision where we share our experiences as peers and we get deputy supervision. I've got two supervisors – one as a family therapist/psychotherapist and an external supervisor on the EMDR treatment.

I find the work here interesting and stimulating. But it is also difficult. We will always offer each client our best efforts. We give them time. We try and sort out any other issues in their life so that they are able to get the best from the treatment we offer.

When I am with a young client, I am building a relationship with them. I try to show that I care about them, that I am trustworthy and effective – that together we can make progress so that they can go ahead with their lives.

Patrick Bentley

For more information about Freedom from Torture:

www.freedomfromtorture.org

https://action.freedomfromtorture.org/freedom-torture-donation-page

Freedom from Torture,
111 Isledon Road, London,
N7 7JW

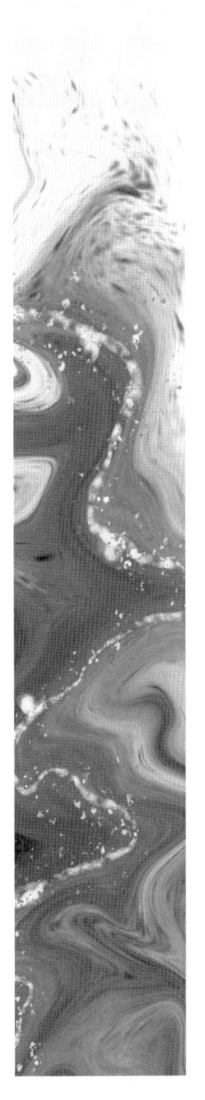

Walking backwards … to savour the moment

In the summer of 2000, along with Barnardo's colleagues and volunteers, I supported a group of families from Glasgow, Edinburgh and Dundee to have a week's holiday at the MacLeod Centre (the Mac) on Iona. Many of the parents and carers were living with addiction, physical and mental health issues, and my work involved providing therapeutic and befriending support to their children in order to help them make sense of, and cope better with, their family situation. The majority of families had rarely been out of their local neighbourhoods, and whilst staying at the Mac was, at times, way out of their comfort zone, it was great to see them begin to experience the magic of Iona.

Among the group was Gary, a nine-year-old boy who came with his mum and stepdad and whose life at home was very difficult due to the chaotic nature of his parents' lifestyles. Being on Iona gave Gary a glimpse of a different kind of world, transforming him from a sad and withdrawn wee boy, to one who was full of smiles and enthusiasm, eagerly jumping at all the activities on offer – arts and crafts, indoor games, outdoor trips, movie nights, daily chores and services in the Abbey – Gary threw himself into the week, each day bringing new experiences and adventures to enjoy. Those around him took delight in his newfound confidence, seeing his innate talents, skills and sense of humour shine through.

Then something happened which burst his bubble … his stepdad had a disagreement with another father, resulting in a physical scuffle and the police having to be called. The atmosphere in the Mac was tense amongst the families, with threats of reprisal, and it was decided that the best thing would be to take the children up to the North End for a walk along the beach. On seeing the water, the children rushed – fully clad, welly boots and all – into the sea with shrieks of delight. Such was the sheer joy of the experience that Gary walked backwards all the way from the North End to the Mac, savouring every moment, taking in a rainbow which appeared with perfect timing.

Sadly, as a result of his stepdad's aggression, it was decided that Gary and his family would have to leave the island, accompanied by the police and one of the volunteers. Gary quietly walked onto the ferry, stood facing a wall and closed his newfound happy persona down, preparing himself, once again, for life back home with his parents.

I continued to work with Gary and his family until I left my job with Barnardo's in September 2002 and was always in awe of his resilience, observing the way in which he switched off his protective shield when I came to collect him, and then switched it back on again when he returned home, finding his own way of managing his parents' rage and mental health difficulties at far too young an age. I thought of him many times over the years and wondered what became of him.

Fast forward to 8 January 2021, 21 years and several jobs later ... and the following e-mail was forwarded by the admin team at my work:

'This is a bit random but I googled Neil Squires ... because he used to be my worker in Barnardo's when I was little, and I was thinking about him the other day so I thought I would Google him and it says he works here. Would there be any chance that you could relay this message on to him, to have his permission to get his e-mail or get in touch with me? I would like to thank him for his help. Understandable this may take some time, because of the pandemic. Thank you, Gary'

A few e-mails and several days later, and I'm sitting chatting via video link to the very same Gary, now 29 years old, and who, given the difficult and challenging childhood he had, is a remarkable survivor. He understandably has his dark days – struggling, at times, with his mental health. His mum sadly died in 2005 and although his stepdad is still alive, he hasn't seen him for years and wants it to stay that way. He has a girlfriend, and is currently studying for an HND in Media and Film studies, having already achieved his HNC. He remembers his time on Iona fondly, and is keen to apply to be a volunteer or maybe visit again. Watch this space!

I like to think that those few days on Iona all those years ago, when he realised people believed in him and he glimpsed a rainbow walking backwards, played a part in helping Gary to keep on walking, and to hope for a time when things would be better.

Neil Squires

Gary

He is walking backwards –
Gary
a small child
with a surprised shock of hair
and a nine-year-old
wonder at the world,
determined
to explore it on his own terms –
walking backwards.

Returning from the shore,
slowly
savouring each moment:
a newborn calf on the croft,
song and smell of the sea,
a crab's claw, a skipped stone,
shared laughter
and the sun chasing the rain …
with a pocket full of shells,
with wave-filled wellies –
walking backwards.

What lies ahead?
Can he help
walking into the sky-darkening squall
of parents' anger?
Where does it leave him –
the violence
of confused and confusing people
confronting death with denial?

Gary,
gazing down the road,
remembering his day,
sees a rainbow over the far shore –
and goes on walking
                        backwards.

Jan Sutch Pickard

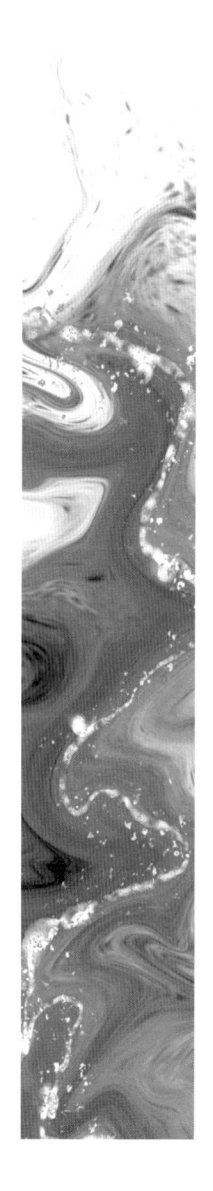

Waiting

Serena and I have been best friends for longer than we haven't. We met aged 11 in high school, and 12 years later we still seek wisdom and laughter from each other.

A few years ago Serena became very ill with the eating disorder anorexia nervosa. She was forced to leave her studies at university to find shelter, healing and peace at home. We all hoped that she would find space to improve her physical and mental condition once she was in close proximity to her family and childhood home.

It wasn't long before it became apparent that it was impossible to plan a nice and simple recovery. Serena deteriorated, which created a hidden but steadily growing sense of panic and frustration in all who loved her. Serena spent thousands of hours talking to therapists, doctors and dieticians.

Nothing seemed to help.

Perhaps inevitably, it became necessary to send Serena to a recovery centre, 145 miles away from home, where she would become an inpatient for an indistinguishable amount of time. There Serena would be cared for 24 hours a day by a pick-and-mix selection of medical professionals, social advisors, therapists, nutritionists, dieticians and trained supervisors. Serena would be placed on a necessarily strict daily regime, with no one but paid strangers to comfort her. As terrifying as the prospect seemed to us, her friends and family, Serena must have felt that dread three-fold. She was finally being forced to face herself, go into a place where all her ultimate fears would be tackled every single day without rest. She was forced to enter the recovery centre with no idea of when she might be discharged, little idea of the realities of what she would face and minimal contact with the outside world.

No one doubted that this was necessary, but the feeling of helpless devastation that this was the reality of Serena's situation was all too powerful. It was like that feeling when you walk up the stairs in the dark, and mistakenly think that there is one more step at the top, only to feel that sickening feeling when your foot falls too far. I felt like I had missed a step in life when Serena was sent away. Just for that moment I was falling, without knowing when the ground would rise up and steady me once again. I will never forget that physical and emotional sensation of watching my best friend being sent away to an unknown place of suffering and fear, and knowing that this was an essential course of action.

The helpless love I felt during that time was unbearable. I would not wish that upon anyone, and yet I know that most people have experienced this feeling in some way. No words can aptly describe the total mix of stomach-twisting, heart-wrenching, fist-clenching emotion I felt when watching my dearest friend manoeuvre through the darkest parts of her life. During this time I felt suspended between grief and hopeful anticipation. Waiting to hear news from anyone. Trying to navigate my own life with Serena still extremely present in everything I did. I was told that Serena's time at the recovery centre would come to an end at some point, but as months began to pass, her discharge seemed no closer. Our waiting refused to end.

On Good Friday, Jesus was put to death in front of all his closest friends. Here, I view Jesus as a man, a son and a friend, not simply as the son of God. Having watched my best friend go through so much pain alone, I may have a small insight into how the disciples might have felt on that day. They watched their beloved friend sent away to a unknown fearful place to experience unimaginable suffering. When Serena was sent away I felt guilt that I had failed her in some way. I cannot doubt that each one of Jesus' disciples felt something similar. At his death, Jesus was within touching distance, and yet, the disciples could do nothing. Disbelief, too, must have plagued the mind of each friend who watched Jesus' death. Just as I asked: how is this happening to my best friend? It cannot be happening because this isn't how I wanted things to happen. This isn't how I imagined things to happen.

It was impossible to tell, in Serena's case, if what we had stretching out before us was indeed a wait, or if it was simply the new reality. Was Serena even going to be discharged, or would she turn into one of those terrible stories where recovery is truly not going to be possible? For Jesus' best friends, those three days must have felt impossible to navigate. Those three days belong to the disciples in a way that none of us can claim: we know that Jesus returned, Jesus' disciples did not. Not everything that belongs to us is easy to own, and yet, that doesn't make it any less precious. I would never wish a wait like I experienced upon anyone, but I would not want it removed from my past. During that time I truly learnt what it was to be a friend. I stubbornly tried my best to help Serena see that she wasn't alone in her suffering, although I don't doubt she felt alone more often than she didn't. The odd letter, gift and visit was all I could do. And for the invisible tie of friendship that was more than enough. Jesus' disciples did all they could: perfuming his body, placing it in a tomb and meeting illegally together. They stuck steadfastly together, and that was how Jesus found them, three days after his death.

Waiting is hell. During the wait we may feel that we contribute nothing and nothing we do makes any difference at all. But I was surprised, in hindsight, at how much I did contribute while I felt that way, and only by speaking to Serena have I learnt what a difference it made. The disciples did what they could and, regardless of how they must have felt, it was exactly what they needed to do. I learnt that, for me, helplessness is a feeling and not a fact. I learnt that waiting is anything but easy, and yet it can be so valuable.

Laura Gisbourne

Working therapeutically with young people during the pandemic

Before the pandemic struck in 2020, research was already clearly showing a decline in the mental health of young people. Universities and colleges had record numbers of suicides and college counselling services often had long waiting lists.

The Scottish Government allocated additional funding to address this issue, and colleges such as the one I work for in Inverness were able to take on additional staff. Then the pandemic hit.

I work predominantly with students (Further Education and Higher Education) between the ages of 16-24. The pandemic has had the effect of making life even tougher, particularly for those who already have a mental health diagnosis. Classes for over 12 months now have been predominantly online, with students not knowing or meeting any of the other people in their classes. Some students are trapped in bedrooms in family homes, some are in student accommodation, some are in bedsits. So isolation is a major issue. One young man tells me: 'I know now how I'll feel if I live to being retired. I have not talked to anyone, apart from the woman at the checkout in Morrisons, for two months now.' His family are in mainland Europe, and so he is unlikely to be able to go home in the near future.

Talk of suicide and self-harm is an everyday occurrence. This ties in with a study funded by the Samaritans, the Scottish Association for Mental Health and the Mindstep Foundation which showed that 14.4% of young adults (3077 adults in the study) reported that at least on one occasion in the previous week they had wanted to end their life. This compares with 9.2% in older populations.[1]

NHS mental health teams have also been affected by the pandemic. Referral for a young person under 18 to Child and Adolescent Mental Health Services in the Highlands is currently years rather than months, with some students waiting two years or more for a referral; then, when they reach 18, they move to a similarly long waiting list for Adult Mental Health Services. With less availability for community mental health teams, more and more students are presenting to us with complex mental health needs, particularly trauma (PTSD), panic, and eating and personality disorders.

As a team, we have had to move from a traditional counselling service offering face-to-face sessions in college to developing a stepped model of care that is delivered online. We can now offer a service tailored to the specific needs of individual students, from crisis drop-in services to well-being groups and workshops, single counselling sessions, e-therapy via messaging and e-mail and longer series of therapeutic sessions where needed. We regularly receive referrals from GPs and where possible work in liaison with Community Mental Health teams. We are, however, a college service, so if students are too unwell to continue with their studies, they are in danger of dropping out of access to mental health care.

There is no evidence to support the theory that mental health of young people will improve as we move out of the pandemic. If anything, as we move from crisis management to resuming everyday life, we are likely to see more mental health distress.

The focus over the last 12 months has, for very good reasons, been on physical health. However, if we do not resource our mental health services to at least have parity with medical health provisions, we will be faced with a crisis which will lead to many more lives lost. The mental health charity Mind is currently running a post-Covid-19 campaign, 'Our Five Tests for the UK Government', asking the UK government to:

– *Invest in community services.*
– *Protect those most at risk.*
– *Reform the Mental Health Act.*
– *Provide a financial safety net.*
– *Support children and young people.*

To find out more and to join the campaign, go to: www.mind.org.uk

Susan Dale, written during lockdown

Note:

1. *British Medical Journal,* 21 October, 2020

A young man

When I was working as a mental health support worker, I used to visit a young man living in a tower block in a rough area of Edinburgh. We'd just sit and drink tea and talk. His flat had been broken into three times. He'd been beaten up by a gang who said he was gay ... Every day was hard. He'd had a job, long ago, in a museum, but had a nervous breakdown, and ended up homeless; then 'trapped in the system'.

He did a lot (on top of the list of all the plain, everyday things) just to survive. One thing he'd do was go to charity shops and buy cheap reproductions of paintings with a portion of his giro money. His flat was full of masterpieces – Monets, Van Goghs, Michelangelos, Seurats, Chagalls, Vermeers, Rembrandts ... Underneath, the walls were peeling and water-marked; punched and kicked in by previous tenants. The walls out in the corridor were all graffitied, and echoed when you walked in them: like the building was vacant of soul; there were needles and syringes and empty bottles lying in corners. He'd burn incense in winter to cover up the mouldy-damp smell in his flat. The smell of incense helped 'put him in a better place', he said.

Another thing he'd do was go to the Hermitage, a woods nearby. He explained that some days he felt 'too surrounded by concrete and greyness'. He'd go sit in the cathedral of trees for a few hours. Walk the quiet paths. Look at the wildflowers.

When I asked him why he collected paintings, and took walks in the Hermitage, he thought a moment, and said: '… It's the way I keep hope alive.'

Neil Paynter

The path

I've walked this path many times before, the crunching of branches beneath my feet. The scuffs on my shoes that show the wearing of time. The smell of decaying foliage sweeping across the path's floor. The wind harsh against my face and no sign of the sun anywhere to be found. The aching inside of me telling me to turn back and wondering why I am here.

But this time it's different, it feels strange and new.

The ground is soft below and the scuffs on my shoes don't appear so noticeable. The wind caresses my cheeks and brings with it a sweet smell, a smell of life, of flowers in blossom and of damp earth waiting to harbour new life.

Above me I see light pouring through the trees, flooding the path with all of its earthly colours. The birdsong around me is flowing through my body and is calling me to follow further in. The aching has gone, replaced with a feeling that this experience is a sign of new beginnings and the start of something great.

This is the path I should be on.

Katie Frost

David's story

A story from a friend …

I used to smoke a lot of weed. This was back in the days when I was feeling really depressed and stressed out. Back in my early 20s. I'd dropped out of university and had no idea what to do with my life. I had a job in a video store: videos were big back then. I worked in the evenings, got home around midnight, and sat up and smoked weed and watched videos.

I smoked weed and watched movies all night, then crashed, and got up and went to work. The job wasn't hard; I didn't have to be too 'with it'. I'd spend all my time doing that. I thought about going back to school but had no money. And no ambition or direction anyway. I lived in a tiny apartment.

Smoking weed took me away from thinking about my future, about my girlfriend, who'd broken up with me, and about some heavy-duty family problems I couldn't deal with then. Made me feel mellow and detached from things. I'd watch movies like *Star Wars* and *The Wall*. Or put music on my stereo and listen to it in headphones, and get lost deep in a landscape …

One day I went out to meet my connection, who had a good regular supply of Colombian, but missed him somehow, and somehow ended up in the middle of a sort of woods nearby. I glanced around, and thought it would be a cool place to come and smoke weed sometime. I sat in the forest, on this crumbling log … I heard the birds singing. Gazed at the pattern of light and shade. I liked the space. It was sort of calming. I went back some days. Sometimes I brought weed along; sometimes I didn't.

The more I went there, the more it felt like *my* place. Not that I grew possessive of it, but I got to know it, explore it. I noticed different birds, and went home and looked them up in a book I'd bought. I went there in different seasons – saw the technicolor autumn; and in the springtime, the buds coming out; little red berries in wintertime, with the scent of spruce and pine. In the summer, I even picked some blueberries. And ate them. There was something about being there. I felt more connected. Rooted. I felt less lost in the forest of my self; less trapped in the tangle of Me.

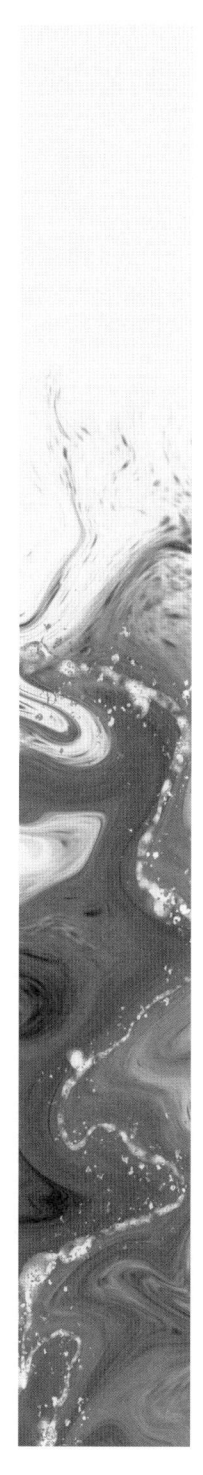

One day I went, and found some company there, starting to cut the woods down. I asked them what they were doing. 'Cutting the woods down to build more houses,' they said. 'You can't cut the woods down!' I said. 'Just watch us,' the guy said, and revved up his chainsaw.

I was angry. I called up the local council. They said there had been a community consultation, months ago, and it was all decided: the resolution was passed and I couldn't do anything about it. I was furious. 'Well, then call Greenpeace,' the woman said, and hung up.

So I did! I talked to someone at Greenpeace, and they sent me some information on the destruction and loss of green spaces in cities and urban areas. They said I probably couldn't do much about the woods now, but there were other things I *could* act on before it was too late. There were even worse situations: in Brazil the rainforests were being cut down and the natives of those forests being uprooted or killed – a whole ancient way of life vanishing, and amazing animals and healing plants becoming extinct. They said there was a talk about it at a community centre in town, so I went along. At the meeting they said they were looking for volunteers. So I volunteered.

I felt energised by the work. I found that volunteering during the day, I didn't smoke as much weed. I met some good people; made some new friends.

I got to know a lot about the issues – I'd always liked reading. One day a job opened up at the office, and I applied and got it. I quit the video store and went to work for Greenpeace!

We had a weekend away. A staff bonding thing. A Native American elder led a workshop. He spoke about our relationship to Mother Earth. In our job of protecting the planet we needed to deepen and nurture our connection with Mother Earth, he said. He spoke about the intricate wonder of the natural world, and about the Great Spirit. He spoke about a lot of things I'd felt in the woods but couldn't put into words.

At the end of the weekend, he invited us all to come and sit together in a sacred circle, and to take part in a healing ceremony. As part of the ceremony, he burned a braid of sweetgrass. Sweetgrass was a gift of Mother Earth, he said. 'The hair of Mother Earth.' We all came from the womb of Mother Earth, he said.

It smelled a bit like weed – but nicer. More like incense. He passed it around the circle. He said to fan the smoke over your heart ... and then over your mind ... and then over your entire body ... I did. And felt different after. More whole.

I've since gone back to university. I'm studying environmental law. It'll be a long road but I'll get there. I want to do everything I can to protect Mother Earth.

To support myself while I'm studying, I work on environmental documentaries. I do research, even write some scripts – so I guess all that experience in the video store and watching all those movies all night didn't go to a total waste!

Neil Paynter

A child at heart
Luke 18:17

One Christmastime, years ago when I was working as an aide in a nursing home, I asked a lively 96-year-old woman, who I was sitting with helping to eat, the secret of a long life. 'A glass of sherry before bed,' she answered, and I laughed ... 'Believe it or not, I still feel like a child at heart ... Otherwise, it's hopeless,' she said seriously. It suddenly felt like it was she who was feeding me.

Like the old woman in the nursing home, I still feel like a child at heart. Sometimes in an immature way – I feel frightened, insecure, needy ... But at other times, I feel a childlike sense of wonder and joy – and I'm suddenly able to be silly, to laugh, to dance. And it feels like a healing flood of God's infinite grace and love.

At another time, I taught English as a second language to adults and children. One afternoon (when we were covering verbs, I guess), I wrote this on the blackboard for the children to fill in with whatever words they liked: SOMETIMES I'M HAPPY _____.

Sometimes I'm happy

Sometimes I'm happy standing in the summertime blue
Sometimes I'm happy talking to you

Sometimes I'm happy dancing the spin-around-dizzy
Sometimes I'm happy sitting still in the busy

Sometimes I'm happy waving to train people
Sometimes I'm happy leaping
my mind off the steeple

Sometimes I'm happy
playing my harmonica
(but my cat isn't)

Sometimes I'm happy wearing my straw hat all day
Sometimes I'm happy watching my cat at play
(or watching my cat
knead and purr,
knead and purr the comforter)

Sometimes I'm happy talking to cows, and crows

Sometimes I'm happy taking I'm-the-most-famous bows

Sometimes I'm happy eating macaroni and chocolate sauce

Sometimes I'm happy using the good cups for tea

Sometimes I'm happy grabbing Babshe's ears
Sometimes I'm so happy I'm in tears

Sometimes I'm happy swinging my self

Sometimes I'm happy running where I wanna get
Sometimes I'm happy meeting someone new I've never met yet

Sometimes I'm happy seeing the bottom – then a fish
Sometimes I'm happy squishing and stirring
ice cream in a dish

Sometimes I'm happy seeing something very small
(like a tiny red spider)

Sometimes I'm happy saying favourite words, like 'mariposa'

Sometimes I'm happy collecting stuff
(like shells and rocks and coins,
and house and car keys people have lost in grassy fields
and car lots)

Sometimes I'm happy how the way geese fly and honk

Sometimes I'm happy hearing a banjo
plink
plank
plunk …
flaillllll

Sometimes I'm happy for no reason at all –
and I think that's the happiest happy of all

Write your own 'Sometimes I'm happy' poem …

Neil Paynter

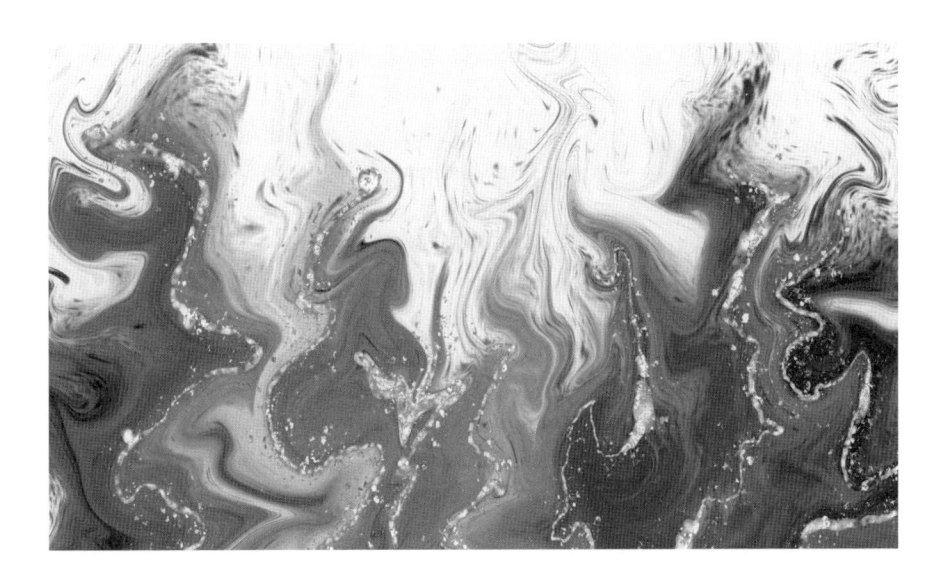

Older people

Holy ground

It was a beautiful Sunday afternoon. The sun was shining brightly as we set off to visit my favourite auntie. These visits were always bittersweet because Auntie was suffering from dementia and now lived in a residential home.

Over the previous two years we had watched as she had become increasingly confused, forgetful and mentally frail. Always a good cook, Auntie had lost the ability to follow recipes, remember what ingredients she had already used and what else she still needed to add. Dinner was served with 'some little round, green things and those long, orange things'. After she was widowed there was increased concern. The Home help often noticed an almost empty fridge and little evidence of meal preparation. Auntie had also been seen wandering near a busy road, unsure of how to get home. Social Services decided that she needed to go into a care home, but Auntie was unwilling to leave her bungalow. Admittedly, hitting the social worker with her handbag was not the smartest reaction, and so this frightened elderly lady was sectioned under the Mental Health Act.

Eventually we had found her a place in a residential home run by the Salvation Army. It was homely and caring. Food was well-cooked, there were gardens to sit in and it was situated in a village nearer our home. We were certain Auntie would be well-cared-for and hoped she would be happy there.

There were, of course, the inevitable pleas to come and live with us – 'I won't be any trouble' – or requests to find a little house where she could look after herself. There were tears, and occasionally mini tantrums, as we struggled to explain why these were not options. There were laughs, too, as Auntie looked at my husband, and then at me. 'I could do with a good man,' she said. 'Do you have any more like him at home?' 'Afraid not,' I answered. 'Just the one!' 'Oh well,' Auntie replied, 'just thought I'd ask!'

It did not seem fair, when Auntie had devotedly cared for her parents for many years, that she could not be cared for by her family, but we had lived through six years of gradually saying 'goodbye' to my mother-in-law, so we knew the score; and we also knew our limitations.

We created a memory book – photographs of family and friends, programmes of the many shows Auntie had appeared in, and some views of the town where she had lived most of her life. Her response was one of fleeting interest. Once a gifted artist, Auntie was no longer interested in painting. She said she did not know how to do it any more. We soon had to accept that the talented, vibrant and fun-loving lady we had known for so long was gradually disappearing and retreating into a world of her own. Conversations were becoming more difficult too, so we usually communicated through hugs, touch and smiles.

That Sunday afternoon at the home, Auntie decided that she'd like to stay for the short worship service, so I agreed to keep her company. Many of the residents had been Salvation Army officers and dressed in their uniforms for the occasion. Physically and mentally frail they may have been, but their spirit and faith were obviously still strong. One lady stood up, sauntered across to the piano bench, opened the lid and rifled through the music inside before closing the lid with a loud bang and wandering back to her chair. This was going to be interesting! The officer-in-charge announced a hymn and read the words of the first verse. I opened the hymnbook at the right page and handed it to Auntie, even though I was unsure if she could still read. It wasn't a hymn I recognised. Suddenly Auntie squeezed my hand and gave me a big, beaming smile. 'Isn't that lovely?' she asked. I looked around the room wondering if she had noticed a flower arrangement or a picture.

'No, the words,' she told me. They were about the love of God for each of us.

When it came to the Lord's Prayer, Auntie was word-perfect and confident. I was amazed.

This was a lady who was increasingly unable to communicate verbally with any of us. I felt as Moses undoubtedly did when he saw the burning bush. It was a completely unexpected and incredible experience of God's presence. In spite of the faint smell of urine occasionally wafting round the room, surely this was holy ground?

A Dutch lager company had been running a series of amusing adverts on TV. They claimed that their superior product could reach the parts other lagers could not. This unexpected experience of God's Spirit at work seemed to be the spiritual equivalent. Proof that even when an illness such as Alzheimer's has reached the stage where it is a struggle for sufferers to communicate verbally, that God's Spirit still can – and does – reach them.

Years earlier, Auntie had bravely taken me and a friend to Paris before our A-level exams. We had been given details of the morning service at a mission church on the outskirts of the city. (Someone my dad knew who worked there had organised our accommodation.) Auntie was not enthusiastic because she was not a regular churchgoer but decided it would be rather bad manners not to go. It was Easter Sunday morning and the joy which erupted during the last hymn – 'À toi la gloire, O Ressuscité!' – was almost tangible, even if you could not understand French. Little was said afterwards. However, when we knew Auntie was dying we opened the instructions she'd written down for us several years previously; there it was: the final hymn she had chosen for her funeral was 'Thine be the glory, risen, conquering Son!'

Kathy Crawford

Nurse's notes

Extracts from a longer piece about working as a nurse's aide

Amazing Grace

Jane is far away in her interior landscape. She sits in her room all day. Locked in a wheelchair. Hums and sings to herself. Loudly sometimes, as if saying: 'I'm still here. I'm *still* fucking here.'

There's a piano in the unit. I played 'Amazing Grace' – and Jane sang along.

Amazing how someone who can't remember their daughters' and sons' and spouse's names can remember all the words to some old song. Music is holy. Music is the voice of God.

I played Jane 'Summertime'. And she sang along – her voice rough and broken and sore and beautiful. Tears in her throat.

Suddenly a joke about chickens

People can seem so disoriented – calling out for the dead. Then suddenly start reciting a poem they learned in grammar school, word for word; or, out of nowhere, suddenly start telling you a joke about chickens:

'Farmer buys two chickens and puts them in his basement, and weeks pass and he has a whole bunch of chickens. Flock … Yeah, but then it rains and the basement floods and they all drown one night.

'So, he calls up his alderman and says: "I bought chickens and now they've all drowned."

'And the alderman says: "I can't do anything, call the mayor."

'So the farmer calls the mayor and says, "I bought chickens and now they've all drowned – what am I supposed to do?" And the mayor says, "Geez, I'm sorry, try the president, try the President of the United States."

'So the farmer calls the President, and the President says: "I can't do anything, my hands are tied. Next time buy ducks."'

Elma

Sitting in the dining room, trying to help Elma eat:

'I can't eat, I'm dead, oh, please, no.'

'… You can't eat because you're dead?'

'Yes … I can't even pick up that glass there.'

'You can't pick it up because it's too heavy? … You can't pick things up because you're dead?'

'Yes. I'm hollow inside. I'm living in a dead body.'

'Your body is giving out on you.'

'I'm dead. See, I can't pick it up – I wish someone would believe me.'

'Because you're dead everything is so heavy?'

'Yes.'

Paul

'Everyone's dead,' says Paul. 'Everyone's dead up here, you know,' and I look around at everyone staring with fish eyes and see what he means.

'But you're not,' I say. 'You're not, Paul – you're full of spirit yet.'

'You bet cha. You bet cha!' And he eats everything on his plate. Has me scoop up the crumbs.

Paul was in the war. Afterwards, played guitar and harmonica and rambled round. Then settled down and farmed.

I push him back to his room after lunch. He can't sleep any more, he tells me. Just ten or fifteen minutes at a time. Like he's afraid of going to sleep and waking up dead.

During the afternoons he likes to just sit and think, he says. To just sit, and look at his photos up on his wall.

Paul lost his arms somehow. Housekeeping keep piling his clothes and blankets and soaker pads on his nightstand – blocking his view of his pictures. He curses and shakes his head. I pick up the stack and move it out of the way for him. Set it on his bed.

He smiles – cries out because he can suddenly see the vista of his life again. There are framed photos of his dashing older brother who was in the Air Force and got shot down 'too young, too young' …

'I guess any age is too young,' I say.

'You bet cha. You bet cha.'

His wife riding a pinto horse: beautiful, smiling cowgirl with a lasso.

'Well, she sure lassoed me,' Paul says.

He and his army buddies who got killed, or else lost on the way …

I leave Paul with his memories and thoughts.

'Thank you!' he calls. 'Thanks.'

Grace

We're dolling everyone up for the Christmas party. Putting on make-up. Giving manicures. I grab an emery board, and sit and file and shape Grace's thick yellow fingernails that have been soaking … We have a good chat.

'And so what about a little Christmas glitter on those nails, Grace?'

'Oh, no thanks, dear – I've never been the flashy type.'

Everyone is having a good time. I give Grace a facial. Smooth and massage Pond's Cold Cream into her tired, dry wrinkles. She closes her eyes – it must feel good. I wonder how long it's been since anyone has touched her (not counting turning her to change her, not counting wiping her rear). I wonder if she remembers a lover; a son; the summer breeze – fragrant as Pond's Cold Cream.

Home

I visit Vera in her bedroom. She sits in her chair, with her 'posture pal'.

'Hello, Vera!' I call. 'So how are you today?' …

She sits gazing. Out the window. In at the past. Chants rhythmically at intervals: 'Are-e, Are-e, Are-e, Are-e …' – to stimulate and comfort herself I guess. 'Are-e, Are-e, Are-e …'

I touch her arm … Make eye contact.

'Oh, hello,' she says, and smiles. She tells me that she's sitting waiting for Philip to come and take her home. 'Are-e, Are-e, Are-e, Are-e …'

I ask her who Philip is and she tells me her brother.

'Your little brother?'

'Are-e, Are-e, Are-e … I think so. I want to go home in the worst way. I want to go home in the worst way now. Are-e, Are-e, Are-e, Are-e …'

'Is Philip at home?'

'Are-e, Are-e, Are-e, I guess he'd be home now. At the house.'

'… What kind of house? What kind of house is it?'

'Not a big house, but it's a nice house. Are-e, Are-e, Are-e, Are-e …'

'A nice house.'

'Nice house … Warm … I wanna go to my bed.'

'Warm like your bed?'

'Yes … Are-e, are-e, are-e. Not a lot of rooms but a nice house. Flowers.'

'Flower gardens?'

'Yes … Are-e, Are-e, Are-e, Are-e. It's way out in Hanover. I'm Hanover. It's outside of Hanover. I want to go home in the worst way. I want to go home in the worst way now.'

'To the nice warm house with Philip.'

'Yes … I wish Philip would come and take me home. So, I sit and wait for him. I sit and wait for him to take me home. Are-e, Are-e, Are-e …'

Everyone here longs to go home. Home to their home – their real home. Home to the past. Home to their mother and father. Home to their brothers and sisters. Home to their husbands and wives and children. Home from here, from this place called a home. Home to God. Home to Mother earth. Home to the universe.

They wander up and down the long, narrow hallways, searching for a way out, a way home. The doors are locked.

'Are-e, Are-e, Are-e, Are-e …'

Neil Paynter

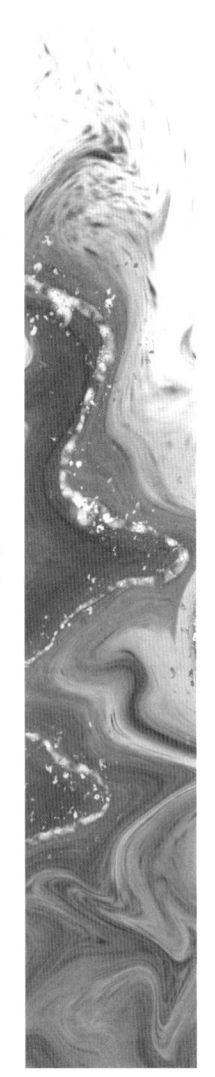

It smells like loneliness

Gordon lived in the same seniors apartment building as my grandmother. One afternoon when I was over helping my gran with her Christmas decorations – out in the hallway hammering her wreath up on her door – Gordon came out and asked me if I could please help him put up *his* decorations one day. He didn't want to get himself all upset, he said ...

The TV and radio are conversing loudly when I come in ...

Gordon's apartment is crowded with knick-knacks: figurines, mugs with faces; things from the house he didn't have the heart to part with, framed photographs of his mother ... Gordon gets me a Labatts Blue from the fridge, which is bare except for bottles of beer. He's got some leftover Chinese food from the Pomegranate heating up on the stove, on low.

He's relieved that I'm here to do the lights and decorations because he doesn't want to get himself all upset. Last year he did it all by himself and he got so upset. 'I'm too old,' he says. 'I've made my mind up – I'm not getting myself upset any more.'

He's got a white plastic tree, a garland he bought today over at the Home Hardware, a set of those little blinky white lights, tangled frustratedly in a box ... I get working on it.

'Take a beer break,' he says.

The tree goes up pretty easily, after I figure it out. In a rush of Yuletide inspiration, I duct-tape the garland up around his fake fireplace.

'Oh gosh – I'm just thrilled with that!' he exclaims. 'I just love how you've draped it around like that. That's wonderful. See – if I was doing it, I'd be so upset by now. Here, have a beer.' (I'm still working on the first one.)

I sit down for a moment, and glance around the apartment. He must have about twenty mobiles hung up: flocks of birds, constellations of stars, butterflies, doves, mobiles made from seashells ... All twisted and tangled.

He started collecting them after his second wife died, he tells me.

'That's another thing I wanted to ask you to do – I'd do it myself but I'd just get upset.'

So I untwist and untangle Gordon's mobiles for him; walk around the two-roomed apartment and free them, one by one.

He reaches over and switches on the ceiling fan, and they all start speaking softly. Chimey ones; soft, gongy ones …

'Oh, I just love this,' he says. 'Sometimes I just sit here and listen. It's so peaceful and calming.'

It's good to see the birds and butterflies and stars swaying and dancing again.

'Have a beer break.'

The duct tape is so old it either doesn't stick at all, or else sticks for a bit then slowly peels away, pulling off paint.

'Oh, don't worry about it,' Gordon says. 'What's a little paint? It doesn't matter. Nothing like that matters in life – believe me!'

As I untangle the lights, and hang them up around the fireplace with the garland, Gordon tells me about the last Christmas he spent with his mother. 'I was just sitting here remembering,' he says.

He visited her Christmas Eve: she was up at the nursing home by then.

'It was the best place for her … I asked the nurse if it would be all right if I brought her some liquor in. "Sure, why not?" she said. It was a lovely green colour. I forget what it was now, but this lovely green colour. I had glasses, beautiful glasses I brought along. We sat in the big room that they have there, by the big window, and just watched the snow fall together, and drank a couple glasses. Lovely … Then the nurse came by and said, "You have to go back to your room now." So, we went back and had one more glass there. Then I put mother to bed. Lovely. I always remember it. Especially now at Christmastime.'

He was adopted, he reveals. 'I think of my adopted mother as my real mother,' he tells me.

The TV's turned down now with just the picture: The Community Listings: … A country square dance somewhere … The Distress Line.

Easy listening on the radio. 'The relaxing, mellow sounds of WEAZ.'

Gordon asks me what I'm doing for Christmas.

I tell him that I'll be with family.

He'll be here, he says. Enjoying the decorations.

And on Christmas Eve he'll go and visit the woman who used to work as his mother's maid. She's deaf and dumb, but can read lips. She lives just outside of town. He takes a cab over and checks in on her from time to time. Last year she came over and he made a turkey with all the fixings. Cranberry sauce. This year they're going to keep it simple. She gave him the embroidery there on the wall. The papier mâché cat beside the television.

'We're friends. She loved mother, and we've known each other such a long time.'

I finish the decorating. As I'm packing away the boxes, Gordon asks me if I'd like to order a pizza, his trembling, arthritic hand on the receiver. I thank him very much but tell him that I really have to get home.

'Well, I've got my Chinese food heating.' It smells like loneliness.

'Another beer then?'

'One for the road.'

I plug in the lights and we sit together a moment; he switches off the high light.

'Oh, now that's just beautiful! I just love the way you draped it around like that. Now I can just sit here and look at it and enjoy it without getting upset.' And underneath, the mobiles make soft, gentle, sad sounds …

I get up to go. Gordon pulls himself up to say goodbye, and reaches in his pocket for his wallet and holds out 50 dollars. 'No, here, take it, it's worth it. It's worth it not to get upset.'

I explain I can't – I've only been there a couple hours. Not even. I accept fifteen. 'We're friends,' I say.

He smiles.

I leave, feeling not so much drunk but overloaded with life.

My gran dies in the New Year, but I help Gordon with his decorations for a couple more Christmases, until he moves into a nursing home. I visit him there at Christmas once; sneak some whisky in. We sit and watch *It's a Wonderful Life* on the common room television.

The next Christmas I come again, but he doesn't know me any more. I leave the home, and walking down the dark country road gaze up at the night sky, tangled with stars.

Neil Paynter

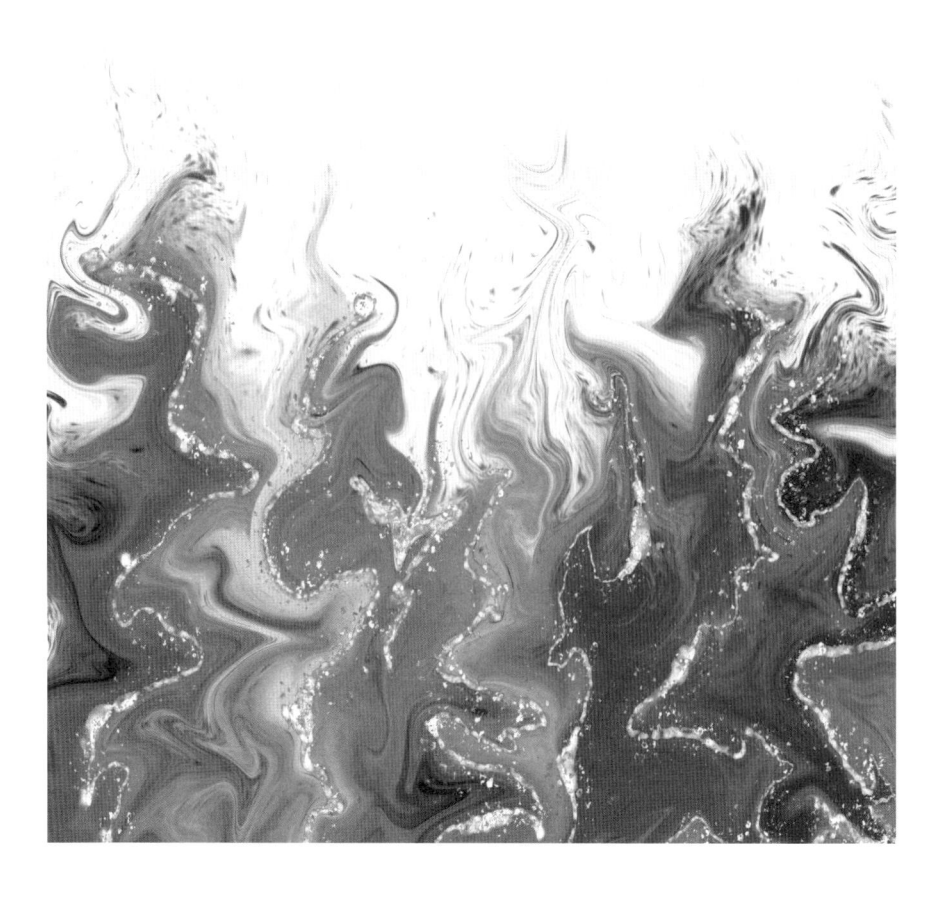

Well-being

Burnout

Burnout is a common experience of those involved in caring work, such as ministers, doctors, nurses, teachers, social activists ... Often conflated with stress and depression, it is related to but not the same as either.

The symptoms of burnout can be seen as defence mechanisms – a way of shutting down and disengaging when life has become too painful. People who are stressed are caught up in over-engagement (although this may precede burnout as we try harder to cope and fix all the problems). In the stressed state we tend to overreact emotionally; burnout is associated more with feeling numb. Stressed people tend to recover from the emotional and physical trauma once they are able to de-stress. In burnout, the primary wounding is emotional and spiritual and tends to linger even if stress has diminished and physical well-being has recovered. The cause of stress can usually be pinpointed and can come and go quickly as the stress source is present or absent. Burnout tends to have a more gradual onset (often the cause is obscure), and gradually worsens until crisis point when the person can barely function at all, even if the apparent cause of the stress is withdrawn. Burnout tends to produce a sense of hopelessness, helplessness, loss of ideals, fear, demoralisation, while the focus of stress is more on disintegration and inability to function. Burnout produces a depression rooted in turning inwards to protect oneself, whilst depression with stress is a way of coming to a halt in order to restore energy and vitality.

The roots of burnout lie in a loss of sense of being in right relationship with ourselves, significant others in our lives and our work. We can feel alienated from a workplace that does not 'walk its talk' – for example having an ethos of caring for others yet overloading and failing to care for those it employs. At the personal level, we can feel out of balance, doing work or being in relationships that are no longer true for us.

Burnout predominantly affects professional carers who may be bringing their natural heartcentredness into their jobs. In doing so they seem to get into patterns of over-giving while under-receiving – valuing looking after others but often neglecting to value themselves. One of the solutions to burnout is to move more to patterns of equally valuing the caring of the self: feeding one's own soul as much as that of others. This requires us to explore why we have become caught up in over-giving, in controlling or co-dependent relationships in caring work, in an excessive 'neediness' to care and its rewards; why we have difficulty in knowing and maintaining healthy relationships and boundaries for ourselves.

Work and caring pressures are factors in burnout it is true, but these are often the agents provocateurs rather than the root causes. Burnout is the desperate cry of the very essence of who we are/the highest self/the soul to break free. It is symptomatic of a longing to be liberated, no longer defined by who or what others say we are. It is the struggle to be in the world in which we find and give love and compassion; have work and relationships that have heart and meaning for us. It is the longing to be free of old wounds and other unconscious processes that limit our definitions and understanding of ourselves, our freedom to be in the world fully and authentically who we truly are. This struggle for truth and authenticity, when we are trapped in work and relationships that inhibit or edit us and which no longer nurture us, can lead to an experience of profound exhaustion. It is an exhaustion made worse by confusion if we can see no way out, or don't understand why we feel so bad, or try to help ourselves by injecting even more effort to get things back to 'normal'.

Burnout is a spiritual crisis in the sense that it goes to the very roots of where we find meaning, purpose and connection in life. Everything that we once thought of as normal or valuable or certain in our lives can suddenly be thrown into turmoil. We can feel trapped by impossible demands, spiritually arid, hopeless, faithless and empty.

The spiritual aridity of burnout is a form of deep human suffering at every level (physical, psychological, social, as well as spiritual) when old ways of being in the world fail and disintegrate. We pour energy into trying to shore up 'normality' but this only makes us increasingly depleted, exhausted and heartsick with the effort. Things seem to fall apart – one thing after another goes wrong.

Disease (dis-ease) in many forms can occur; some can become so distressed that severe physical or mental illness, even suicide, can result.

The suffering is accentuated because the cause is not clear to us (although we may attribute it to external things like work) and our usual resources for dealing with such distress do not seem to work, and we feel like we are in a spiralling, downward struggle demanding more and more effort just to keep functioning; these demands in turn fuelling the burning out, the loss of energy at every level. The vision of a life without suffering eludes us, so we can become immobilised – unable to move to the future while struggling frantically to hold to the painful present. Nothing less than a complete transformation in our way of being is called for, but the prospect of this too can be terrifying. The levels of fear, panic, pain and distress in our lives are often unprecedented.

Tinkering with stress relief has little impact. A thorough assessment by a spiritual director, therapist or doctor, enlightened in the ways of burnout, can be really helpful in getting us to see more clearly what is going on amidst the fog of our own perceptions.

A priority is to pull out of the situation. It might be necessary to take sick leave or move to the home of a friend or to another space where we feel safe and taken care of, or to a specialised retreat centre. Seeking support from a GP knowledgeable in burnout (without this there is a risk of getting a diagnosis of depression) can be helpful, not least because the GP can aid us to see aspects that we might not see ourselves and can sanction sick leave.

Burnout is not a time for action and grasping at solutions – the effort involved can make things worse; this is a time to come to stillness, to recuperate and re-energise, rest and reflect, wait and see; to get out of the situation and find the space and guidance that will allow the solutions that are waiting to emerge from within. We need time and support to reconnect with ourselves and the world, to get access to insight about what has been going on for us, where the roots of the pain lie and how to transform them.

Renewal through burnout is about re-birthing ourselves into the world, about living more authentically with what has heart and meaning for us, living from a place of essence, of soul. For most people this is a time of renewal of relationship not only with self and others, but also with God, where we may find new possibilities of depth and connection become available to us that had hitherto been hidden.

Burnout is a wake-up call to transformation, both personal and organisational.

The right kind of help from the outset means that we can heal through it and reignite, finding new passion and zeal in our lives.

Stephen G Wright

A Holy day

A soul can become dry and brittle like a leaf cut off from its tree-ness. A parched soul will believe it is abandoned on an island in a cold universe; alone, confused and sick of the life that seems intent on destruction of all beauty and innocence. For this soul all wonder has vanished. There is no energy left for inspiration, no ears to hear the revelation of birdsong, no eyes to witness the awe of sky. Only the incessant replay of mind's miserable chatter, hurling itself from past to future and back again, compiling lists of things left undone, words given and received from unhealed wounds and prophecies of doom that furnish a fragile future.

This soul needs a Holy day, a week of Holy days, where it can soak in the sea of being, can rest in the light of non-doing and can sink its roots into the quiet ground of life. Sinews of soul that have been cleaved away from the nourishing source of life need space where time must not be counted. Space to re-member, re-assemble and re-mind the soul of its magnificent rarity. To allow soul muscles to amass, they must be bathed in a forest of rest while the small whittering mind is settled with stories that will smooth the mountains of catastrophe into molehills of gentle peace.

It is all just life, calling you once more to uncover your purpose, to know who you are and draw you into a new dance of freedom and being, free from the oughts and shoulds of an age gone by, into a new time of sensing, seeing and being.

> *Take time now and live in the presence of the present, one breath at a time, and do not worry about tomorrow. Know that not one fragment will be lost without you being found and brought home. Here even the suffering will make sense that only your heart can know.*
>
> *Here the silent strength of life will reveal itself in you and in all that is earth.*
>
> *The sky will remind you of your tiny vastness and of the Presence that cradles you.*
>
> *The clay of the ground which upholds you will re-assemble your bones.*
>
> *The breath that you breathe will re-member its Divine origin and you will awaken again to the mystery in you.*

Bev Robertson

Well-being

For about four years, I convened a committee that was tasked to improve ministers' well-being in the Methodist Church in Scotland. This article includes some of the insights and recommendations we made, which can apply more widely than just to those in full-time church work.

Well-being is a term we can use to describe good mental health. When we use the words mental health there is an immediate association in the contemporary world with mental illness. By using the term well-being we can avoid this unhelpful association. Well-being is truly holistic as it can include physical, mental, emotional and spiritual aspects of a person's life.

Well-being exists when a person is in emotional, mental, spiritual and physical good health and has sufficient energy to meet the demands of their life and work. You will feel good about yourself and your life. You will be curious about what's going on around you, and you will enjoy what you do. The characteristics of well-being are really quite obvious. I list some:

– *contentment*
– *a zest for life*
– *able to laugh and have fun*
– *able to deal with stress*
– *the ability to bounce back after setbacks*
– *a sense of meaning and purpose in life*
– *being flexible and willing to learn*
– *having a healthy life balance including work, rest and play*
– *being able to build and maintain meaningful relationships*
– *feeling self-confident with good self-esteem.*

Very few of us will experience all of these for all of the time but if we fail to recognise any such characteristics in our lives then we probably need to do something about it.

The church often states that ministers are its most valuable resource. If so, they need to be looked after. Worn out and exhausted clergy are not doing themselves any favours and are not doing the church or God any favours either. It is crucial that the church puts structures and systems in place to provide support where needed and helps individuals make beneficial changes to their lives and lifestyles.

Ministers are highly motivated because they have been called by God. There can be no higher motivation, but this can be a double-edged sword.

Look at the poem 'If', by Rudyard Kipling, which many ministers can surely relate to:

> *If you can keep your head when all about you*
> *Are losing theirs and blaming it on you,*
>
> *If you can trust yourself when all men doubt you,*
> *But make allowance for their doubting too …*
>
> *If you can force your heart and nerve and sinew*
> *To serve your turn long after they are gone,*
>
> *And so hold on when there is nothing in you*
> *Except the Will which says to them: 'Hold on!' …*

Though it comes from the very different world of over a century ago, these words still can inspire a spirit of self-sacrificial service. However, such attitudes can also verge on the demonic. Think about the words of the last two lines. Here is a recipe for burnout and heart attacks! Such noble sentiments need to be tempered with Jesus' words reminding us that we have to love ourselves if we are ever to manage to love our neighbours.

Balance in our lives requires juggling, and it seems that today everyone is trying to keep many balls in the air. As we keep our work, health, family, friends and faith spinning, we should recognise that work is a rubber ball and will bounce back if you drop it. All the rest are made of glass – drop one of them and it could be broken or even smashed.

Many things contribute to the well-being of a minister, some of which are in the control of the individual and some of which are in the control of the church. The church plays an enormous role in a minster's life – a much greater role than most secular employers. It is not only employer but also landlord, primary community for day-to-day interaction and setter of moral codes to control your life. It exercises subtle pressure to overwork and has control over family life and choice of home. Such a complex relationship can be good, or it can be very bad.

There are many other negative factors that harm well-being. These include bereavement, loneliness, stress, inactivity, lack of sleep, relationship problems, worries about money or work, poverty or debt and past or present trauma or neglect.

We can counter these negative influences in many ways. Structurally, the church and other employers can put in place systems and support structures to mitigate institutional pressures. There are also many things that an individual can do. Good physical and mental health both require you to stay active, eat well, drink sensibly and experience regular sunlight. We must not be afraid to talk about our feelings and to ask for help when we need it. It is good to keep in touch with friends and cultivate positive relationships. Caring for others or caring for a pet can help. Take time for yourself and do something you are good at. Set yourself a challenge and learn something new, volunteer, take a break, live in the present moment and accept who you are, reframe unhelpful thoughts, and develop gratitude.

Secular commentators point out the value of developing spirituality in a faith community or through an activity like yoga or meditation, and likewise Christians should look to the riches of our traditions for guidance and support. For example, we could say that the Bible tells us that for our emotional well-being, spiritual well-being and social well-being we need love, joy, peace, patience, kindness, goodness, faithfulness, gentleness and self-control. The fruits of the spirit, as identified in Galatians chapter five, are indispensable to wholeness, well-being and experiencing fullness of life.

Working out what triggers stress or poor mental health can help you anticipate problems and think of ways to solve them. If you reflect on events and feelings that could be adversely affecting your well-being, you might be surprised to find out just how much you're coping with.

Many people have demanding jobs and when you're caught up in an exhausting cycle of relentless hours, it's easy to be hard on yourself. Often it is not our boss who gives us a hard time: we do it to ourselves. If you're struggling, give yourself some space. This could mean taking a few days off or getting some support. Once you've taken a step back then you can make more informed choices.

John Butterfield

Loneliness makes you sick

After mum died, it seemed the right thing to do was to go back home and live with my dad. He was lonely and struggling to cope, even to make a meal for himself. Like many working-class men of his time, his role in the home was clearly defined and cooking had never been part of it, likewise paying the bills, shopping and cleaning.

As the youngest and only single child (this was 1971, I was 21), it was assumed by the family that I'd be the one to help dad out, even though I had not lived at home for two years.

We did not get on well before mum's death and we got on a good deal worse afterwards. To avoid the fights, I would spend as much time out with friends or at work as possible, which rather defeated the point of my living with him. He never shared his feelings or his grief, except to say once, 'It doesn't matter who is around, once that bedroom door is shut there's nothing but loneliness.'

I'd fulfilled the role of dutiful son and gone back to live with my dad. Having someone around the house may have abated the loneliness he felt, but my presence was at best a temporary distraction from it. In his heart of hearts he was on his own at a deep level, because the love and connection were not there, either with myself, his wife of 40 years, or anyone else, and he did not believe in a God.

Loneliness and aloneness (solitude) are not the same thing. It is possible to be alone and not feel lonely. It is possible to be among others and feel loneliness.

Loneliness is a psychological and spiritual pain, a sense of disconnection from others, and for some the very Source of life itself. It leaves us feeling without love, support and intimacy. In this subjective experience we feel cut off and apart from other people, even though they may be nearby.

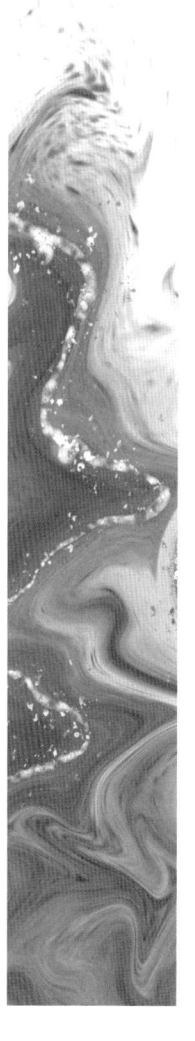

Solitude is a voluntary experience, a choice to be without the company of others for whatever reasons. Our feelings of being connected to or loved by them are not contingent upon their physical presence. For persons of a religious persuasion, where there is a belief in Something Other, complete solitude is impossible anyway. One of the names commonly attributed to the Divine in Judeo-Christian literature is the Presence. If such a Presence is a reality for us, loneliness is arguably impossible, a theme to be developed later in this exploration.

Much of the literature on loneliness focuses on the psychological pain that is its primary symptom. It is seen as a Darwinian evolutionary defence mechanism, designed to make us seek out the comfort and safety of others. What is often overlooked is the spiritual dimension. There is much historical and biblical evidence to show that cutting people off has been used down the ages to punish people, and even cause death.

D'hel, the word for 'fear' in Aramaic, the language which Jesus spoke, has to do, not with the fear of death or pain or punishment, but with the fear of being excluded, driven away and banished from home and family. In pre-modern cultures this was one of the greatest terrors, for there was little opportunity to seek social support elsewhere. People largely lived and died locally within small family and tribal units. To be cast out from this meant the pain of living alone, a kind of social and emotional death, exacerbated by being cut off from the sacred rites, rituals and the presence of the Divine that could only be found in such communities. To be separated from community thus meant separation from God as well.

Nowadays exclusion is still used as a means of control; some religious organisations (such as the Amish or Jehovah's Witnesses) and sects and cults of all sorts will 'shun' people by ignoring them, cutting them off from normal social discourse or family and community connection if they have in some way transgressed the group's rules.

We are human belongings not just human beings. We experience a pain which longs for relief when we are involuntarily cut off from others. For those for whom the Divine is real, then to be cut off from that Source is the greatest and most painful exile of all. Mystical and religious literature across all traditions often expresses the pain of feeling disconnected from the Source. The cry of despair of Jesus in Matthew 27:46 sums this up in words from Psalm 22: *'My God, my God, why have you forsaken me?'*

While short-term loneliness may spur us into seeking connection and association with others, there is abundant evidence that in the longer term loneliness is very unhealthy. The desire not to be alone, or more accurately to avoid the hurt of loneliness, can lead us to participate in relationships or groups that might be harmful to us. One of the responses of those who feel trapped in violent relationships or cults, when asked why they do not leave, is that even an unhealthy status quo is better than the fear of facing life alone.

Many recent studies have shown how loneliness affects health.[1] People who are lonely are more likely to become even more introverted and disconnected from everyday social skills and activities, which in turn creates a cycle of becoming even more socially isolated and unemployable. Lonely people are more likely to place more demands on health and social services, commit suicide, develop lower cognitive function or dementia, have compromised immune systems, and greater risk of heart attacks, strokes, cancer and early death – in fact pretty much any health problem can be said to be exacerbated by loneliness.

Compared to the well-known health hazards of the 'usual suspects' – smoking, lack of exercise, obesity and alcohol consumption – loneliness ranks as an equal, if not greater, health risk. Why might this be so? One factor is the psychoneuroimmunology (PNI) response.[2] Anxiety normally produces a natural defence mechanism in the body – the flight or fight response. Part of this is the readying of the immune system to deal with injury and infection. Normally such a response is transient, as the danger and the associated fear passes. Persistent, low-level anxiety, however, such as occurs in loneliness, seems to have a suppressing effect on the immune system, leading us to be more liable to illness and reduced physiological and psychological resilience.

At the time of writing (January 2021) a Google search of 'Loneliness' produced 375 million responses.

Three quarters of GPs have said they are seeing between one and five people a day suffering with loneliness, and around 200,000 older people have not had a conversation with a friend or relative in more than a month. Government funding has been announced for GPs to use 'social prescribing', which allows them to connect patients with a variety of community-based activities, including cookery classes, walking clubs and art groups. The idea is that it will help people improve their health and well-being, instead of defaulting to medicine.

In universities, figures show that nearly one third (29%) of students experience mental distress, and since 2007 there has been a five-fold increase in the proportion of students with mental health conditions. Often, however, sufferers do not seek help, for there is a social stigma attached to loneliness. Paradoxically this only makes the problem worse – some people try to tough it out or isolate themselves further or pretend that all is well – all of which, of course, heightens loneliness.

Growing awareness of the mental, physical and social problems (and economic costs) produced by loneliness has been accentuated by the infection control demands of the Covid-19 pandemic, including long periods of social isolation for very large numbers of the world's population. Governments and voluntary groups globally have sought to respond to the loneliness impact in the attempt to limit the spread of Covid. Even before the pandemic, government departments in the four countries of the UK had developed extensive policy documents, recommendations and supplied funding to various agencies to help combat loneliness (see Appendix).

In England in 2016, following the murder of the MP Jo Cox, who had a particular interest in the ill-effects of loneliness and its causes, the Prime Minister appointed a 'Minster for loneliness' with a specific brief to explore the causes of loneliness and support initiatives to prevent it. A UK-wide charitable trust (www.campaigntoendloneliness.org) has been set up to identify the causes of loneliness, provide support and campaign for effective strategies to deal with it. It is estimated that there may be as many as nine million lonely people in the UK. Such persons rarely fit the Eleanor Rigby stereotype of the lonely old lady peering through the net curtains. Older people, it is true, are more at risk of loneliness because of the higher likelihood of loss of a spouse or family member, but loneliness appears to affect all ages, classes and races.

Taking a broad view of the many studies into spirituality and well-being, we can suggest that people with the following are more likely to be happy and healthy:

> *Faith – not necessarily in a deity, but simply having faith in something that gives meaning to life – it could be politics, sports or the arts for example, but for most people it is some sort of Higher Power.*

Fellowship – family, friends, community; relationships that cultivate a sense of belonging and being loved.

Fulfilling work that brings creativity, meaning, purpose and rewards and in which there is some sense of autonomy.

Free giving – relationships and voluntary work that provide us with an opportunity to feel that we are giving to others without necessarily expecting something in return.

These '4 F's' in turn help keep another 'F' at bay – Fear – which has detrimental health impacts, for example in compromising the PNI response. More recent groundbreaking studies[3] have shown how the heart is much more than a blood pump, but is its own centre of electromagnetic energy, emotions and consciousness; it is the centre where we feel the sense of love most intensely. Modern science is now demonstrating what the poets, philosophers and lovers down the ages have always known.

It seems that human beings are more dependent on, and realised through, love than any other species. Love overcomes fear. Across a whole range of studies it can be shown that those who receive and give love experience more peace and serenity, health and well-being than those who do not. When that opportunity to feel and offer love is denied, for whatever reason, we experience loneliness, which in turn engenders fear, which in turn makes us sick. Nurturing a sense of fellowship, of loving and being loved, is therefore a counterpoint to the ill-effects of loneliness.

Another dimension of loneliness is that it is sometimes an unconscious experience. We have a sense that something is not quite right in, or is missing from, our lives, but can't quite put a finger on it. Scratch the surface of many behaviours deemed unhealthy and/or socially unacceptable – such as criminality, violence and antisocial behaviour or addictive relationships with drink, drugs, sex, shopping, television and all the other things we may use to get us through the day – and we find that they are tactics we use, rather than to face up to our internal pain. That metaphorical hole in the heart, that lack of human connection, not to say love, brings relentless demands to be filled – with anything, if genuine depth of human contact is not possible for whatever reason.

Curiously, in some studies, the healthiest and happiest people were not those getting support from their religious community, but those who felt they were giving the most. What seems to be going on is that the spiritual-religious paradigm offers people a sense of centre, meaning and connection to others and to the Divine in an often lonely, meaningless and chaotic world.

Our nearest ape relatives spend a great deal of time grooming each other, an act of bonding and strengthening kinship ties, of affirming the place of each member of the group in the hierarchy. We are no less touch and relationship-seeking animals. It may be wondered how far the Covid-19 pandemic has compromised our sense of well-being because of the lack of opportunities to touch each other, to see each other, indeed to see the whole face. To be bonded with others is basic to our survival, to our opportunity to learn who we are as individuals and share in all those relationships and communal activities that help us know what it is to be human.

If loneliness is a problem of disconnection from others, it might at first hand seem relatively easy to solve if we but put the right systems and resources in place to counter it. However, given the complex nature of our longing to belong, simple solutions risk being simplistic and not, literally, getting to the heart of the matter.

Creating and offering access to social clubs and befriending schemes, providing training in computers and Internet access, GPs prescribing social activities – all these, and more, in the recommendations are very laudable. How far they touch in permanent, deep and meaningful ways the lives of those who are lonely is less certain. They may appear to be helpful, but it may be that they are but a temporary occupation of the space that loneliness creates, a distraction from the pain for a little while, until we return to our solitary disconnected state once more.

Remedies for loneliness tend to focus on sticking-plaster options. Arguably there is too little discussion about why societies and communities become atomised and disconnected; about what social structures – schools, clubs, communal activities, etc – we encourage (or discourage). Without the opportunity for authentic bonding, it seems we are at risk of all kinds of faux connections as substitutes, be it demagogic politicians, paranoid groups, which make us feel bonded in our shared paranoia, and all kinds of cults and delusional groups.

For healthy strategies and relationships countering loneliness to work, they have to permit authenticity – they have to feel real to us, rather than a superficial connectedness or receiving the do-goodness help from others. The relationships have to be based on the one thing that join persons together, which is deeper than shared values, politics or occupations – it is the bond that only love can join.

We cannot artificially create relationships just by putting people together. In relating we don't want just anyone. To do so is a mere distraction from loneliness, the fundamental ennui and even despair of existence that only depth of relationship bonded in a sincere affection for one another can heal.

Such a bond, for most people, is more than with people. It seems that for most of us there are limits as to how loneliness can be filled by relationships with persons. A higher bond with the Absolute, whatever we experience that to be, may lie at the root of the longing. God, Goddess, nature, a loving universe, a spirit guide, guru ... any or all of which may help us refute the lie that we are essentially separate.

John Paul Sartre wrote about the *'God-shaped hole'* in human consciousness.[4] But what kind of God? Some imagery cultivates a God who is separate, punishing ... such a God is hardly likely to alleviate a sense of loneliness, or give a sense of being accompanied in love. Those religions that nurture the experience of a loving Presence would seem to offer a remedy for that God-shaped hole, or at least provide a sense of community and fellowship in the pursuit thereof. God and community, or perhaps God *in* community, would seem to offer a substantial solution to the pain of loneliness.

Lockdown has precluded physical connection, but how much worse might it have been without the Internet and its various apps that have enabled people to stay connected in word and visibly? Amid the tragedy, perhaps there has also been an opportunity to reappraise what really matters in life, not least relationships, family and community. And further, as some have argued, to explore more expanded models of family and relationships that support people over and above the model of the conventional nuclear family. The Care Manifesto,[5] for example, urges us to examine the reasons why our societies have become so atomised and how we might reprioritise the direction of public structures, policies and funds into new and revivified old ways of bringing people together and supporting each other along the length of life's journey. Perhaps the pandemic has not so much caused loneliness, as flushed out into the light of day its prevalence from the everyday space fillers that kept it hidden. In being so exposed, amid the suffering, there is an opportunity to look imaginatively at different solutions.

In closing, I am reminded of a conversation I had with one of my greatest teachers, Ram Dass, not long before he died. I'd been exploring loneliness with him, specifically the loneliness that sometimes arose when, as part of a church, I felt unconnected to so much of what was going on and what others believed. It can be very tough if you are mystically inclined to be part of a conventional Christian church, where the emphasis is on believing certain doctrines and adhering to certain stories and practices as absolutes.

In the midst of the conversation, he said, 'You and I have been having this soul-to-soul conversation – what has happened to the loneliness?' Of course my only reply was, 'Gone.' There was something in that depth of conversation that made me realise that the depth of relationship is what transmutes loneliness. We went on to explore that loneliness is entirely an ego concept. The soul is never alone, for it loves, and is loved by, the universe, the Divine. He said, 'I am never alone because I am always with my guru.' Now his guru, Maharaji, had long since left his body. The resolution of loneliness in these terms does not even require the physical presence of the person.

I have spent a lot of my life (in my roles as nurse and spiritual director) alongside people who have been bereaved. I have lost count of the number of times that people have told me, even many years down the line, that although they still miss the bodily presence of the loved one, he or she *'is still with me: I am never on my own'*; there are many studies which report that some people still experience the presence, even the physical presence, of the loved one after their death.

I more deeply understood Ram Dass' comments about his guru, when I came to know my own guru: a long story I have documented elsewhere.[6] Gurus do not have to be with us in body, and that certainly applies to those who know the Presence of Jesus and/or the Beloved. Loneliness seems much less likely to be a problem if we have some form of faith, not just because a faith tends to bring us into social encounters and friendships with others, but also because we recognise the reality of the Something Other, the Presence, the Beloved, in whom and with whom it is not possible to be alone, let alone lonely.

Now, let us extrapolate this to the example of the Iona Community and how the Community may, or may not, counter that painful condition known as loneliness. Like all religious groupings, it brings people together, offering a path of participation and service and communal gatherings large and small, like Community Weeks, plenaries and Family Groups. Membership requires a slow process of induction that includes deepening of relationships with other members, as well as encouragement for members to deepen their individual faith in God. There are communal acts of worship, continued privately in the following of the Rule, which encourages regular reflection and prayer for other members. There is a binding quality to such a community, a strengthening of relationships which mitigates against loneliness – unless of course the participant feels excluded in some way because they do not believe in or cannot adhere to group norms, which is always possible, even with an organisation so apparently open and inclusive as the Iona Community.

The Iona Community is dedicated to the renewal of the church and worship, and is committed to action for peace and justice. Both goals require collective action. The Community brings people together and therefore, almost by accident, contributes to the alleviation of loneliness among those who belong to it. If the Community is doing its job well, the psychological pain that is loneliness is eased by offering connection between participants. The spiritual pain, in those who long for depth of relationship and communion with the Divine, is relieved by the sacred encounter the Community fosters through its religious pursuits. Healthy religious communities have this dual effect upon loneliness – joining us to each other and to the Beloved.

The psychological pain of loneliness is a wake-up call that urges us to look for heartfelt and meaningful connection with persons. The spiritual dimension of loneliness is an equal, if not greater, summons to seek a relationship with the Beloved.

Initiated into this Presence, however we experience it, and in whatever tradition, we may encounter the realisation that we can never be alone and, by extension, never be lonely.

Stephen G Wright, 2021

Notes:

1. For those interested in some of the scientific studies, see the Appendix.

2. *Molecules of Emotion: Why You Feel the Way You Feel*, Candace B Pert, Scribner, 1999

3. *The Heartmath Solution*, Doc Childre and Howard Martin, Piatkus, 2011

4. Quoted in *The Battle for God: Fundamentalism in Judaism, Christianity and Islam*, Karen Armstrong, HarperCollins, 2001

5. *The Care Manifesto, The Politics of Interdependence: The Politics of Compassion*, The Care Collective, Andreas Chatzidakis, Verso, 2020

Appendix:

Some studies on the importance of relationships to and the impact of loneliness on health and well-being:

A Biography of Loneliness: The History of an Emotion, Fay Bound Alberti, Oxford University Press, 2019

'Older adults reporting social isolation or loneliness show poorer cognitive function 4 years later', John T Cacioppo, Stephanie Cacioppo, Evidence-Based Nursing

'Social isolation and loneliness as risk factors for the progression of frailty: The English longitudinal study of ageing', Catharine R Gale, Leo Westbury, Cyrus Cooper, Age Ageing, 2018

'The brain and social connectedness', Eric S Kim, Global Council on Brain Health, 2017

The Lonely Society?, Jo Griffin, The Mental Health Foundation, 2010

'Loneliness predicts increased blood pressure: Five-year cross-lagged analyses in middle-aged and older adults', Louise C Hawkley, Ronald A Thisted, Christopher M Masi, John T Cacioppo, Psychology and Aging, 2010

'The potential public health relevance of social isolation and loneliness: Prevalence, epidemiology, and risk factors', Julianne Holt-Lunstad, Public Policy & Aging Report, 2017

Relationship-Based Care: A Model for Transforming Practice, Mary Koloroutis (Editor), Creative Health Care Management, 2004

'Church-Based Social Support and Mortality', Neal Krause, *The Journals of Gerontology*, 2006

'Recent developments: Suicide in older people', Henry O'Connell, Ai-Vyrn Chin, Conal Cunningham and Brian A Lawlor, BMJ, 2004

'Loneliness and social isolation as risk factors for coronary heart disease and stroke: systematic review and meta-analysis of longitudinal observational studies', Nicole K Valtorta, Mona Kanaan, Simon Gilbody, Sara Ronzi, Barbara Hanratty, BMJ Journals, 2016

Sacred Space: Right Relationship and Spirituality in Healthcare: An Exploration of Right Relationship, Jean Sayre-Adams and Stephen G Wright, Churchill Livingstone, 2000

'Social relationships and physiological determinant longevity across the human life span', Yang Claire Yang, Courtney Boen, Karen Gerken, Ting Li, Kristen Schorpp, Kathleen Mullan Harris, 2016

UK Government website information on loneliness:

Scotland:
https://www.gov.scot/publications/connected-scotland-strategy-tackling-social-isolation-loneliness-building-stronger-social-connections

Wales:
https://gov.wales/loneliness-and-social-isolation-connected-communities

England:
https://www.gov.uk/government/publications/a-connected-society-a-strategy-for-tackling-loneliness

Northern Ireland:
https://www.gov.uk/government/statistics/loneliness-in-northern-ireland-201920

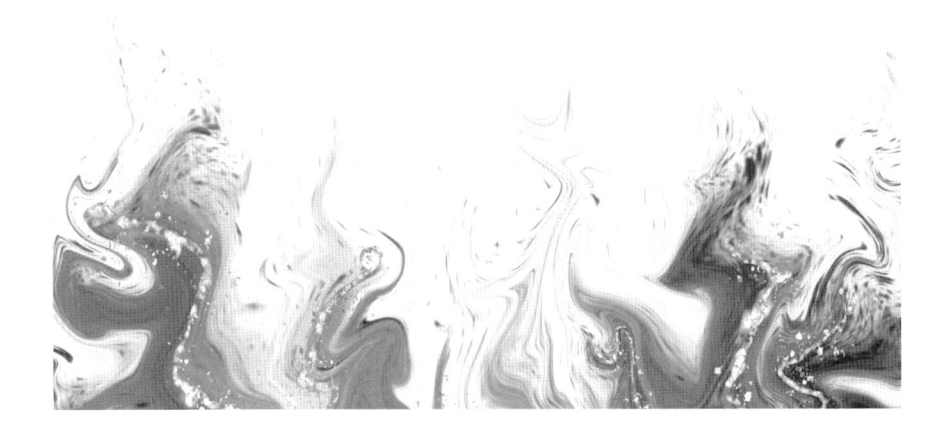

The goodness of nature

Being in nature is one of the best things for my well-being and mental health, and it is widely recognised now by policymakers and service providers as being of great benefit to all. I have been involved in a number of 'green health' projects both as a professional supporting others and for my own personal creativity and health.

Going outside, breathing in fresh air, watching a tree bending in the wind, smelling a flower, feeling the rain land softly upon our skin, placing our hands in the warm earth, listening to the birds or tasting freshly picked fruit are things we often intuitively know are good for us. The stillness, sense of peace and calm that being in nature brings is affirmed both in spiritual wisdom and scientific research. Indigenous communities, healers, shamans, poets and prophets around the world have always shared a deep sense of reverence for nature, founded on a sacred respect for the earth and all beings. One of the most well-known Christian mystics, Julian of Norwich, said that *'The first good thing is the goodness of nature. God is the same thing as nature. The goodness in nature is God.'*[1]

Increasingly, science has supported the value of nature connection; for example, research shows that bacterium found in soil stimulates serotonin production, which improves well-being. The World Health Organisation has presented a report (written by Exeter University) to policy and decision-makers that demonstrates the vital importance of accessible, quality green spaces to physical and mental health.[2]

The development of 'green health' projects and polices has been significant in recent years. Continuing budget cuts to primary and social care have left many people waiting months, or even years, for any kind of psychological help and 'social prescribing' is by no means a replacement for this. However, creating opportunities for people to connect with nature can and does improve a sense of wellness, belonging and purpose and this is well-documented by organisations such as Thrive and Trellis.[3] The theme of 2021's 'Mental Health Awareness Week' was 'nature' and the Mental Health Foundation produced a policy report that showed 45% of people said that connecting with outdoor space enabled them to cope better with the Covid pandemic.[4]

Sadly the opposite is also true, and access to nature is not equitable. Studies show that health outcomes are poorer in those who have less access to greenspace, and time in nature cannot negate structural traumas such as poverty, racism and gender violence. A regenerative culture of genuine equality and sustainability is a radical necessity for the health of the planet and all beings.

As a youth and community worker and activist, both science and spirituality have guided and informed my work over the years, work that has involved supporting vulnerable people to learn to grow veg, use herbs, learn to forage and to experience walks and camps in the wild. One project I initiated was supporting women to learn about and enjoy the environment. Most of them were living in very stressful situations with myriad challenges.

One week we took a trip to a farm, where we did some practical and reflective activities. Some of the women had never been to the countryside and were apprehensive and a little cynical about the trip; gradually they overcame their wariness and visibly began to relax, basking in the sun, throwing sticks on the fire and walking under the canopy of trees as sunshine and shade flickered across their faces. What struck me most was not the 'organised' parts of the trip, but the excitement, playfulness and joy the women expressed when we encountered some lambs, or when we played 'Pooh Sticks', or toasted marshmallows on the fire. On the way back we sang songs and chatted in the minibus: in stark contrast to the silence and nervousness on the way there. It was just one day out in the midst of very tough lives, but the experience helped them and one of the comments on the day was 'I have never felt this relaxed in my life'.

In another job, I was part of a team who took vulnerable young adults to stay in a bothy in true Scottish wilderness. Every one of the young people we took had experienced trauma of some sort. Many of them had been pathologised as 'challenging', or 'difficult', yet they often showed kindness, caring and insight that revealed who they truly were. For many, being out of the city was a new experience – looking at the stars in the clear vast night sky, planting and tending trees, sitting round the fire, cooking for each other all brought a sense of community and connection. They were able to share their skills and gifts: one young man discovered a real talent for drystane dyking, which really built his confidence and self-esteem. Many of the outcomes were quantifiable in terms of increased teamwork skills, a sense of accomplishment, new skills, new friendships, though it was often their comments that revealed the benefits of the experiences. One young person said, 'It's the thought of coming here that stops me going back to the drugs. I imagine being here, with the wind on my face, every time I feel low.' Another comment was 'I love the freedom, people trust us, there's no judgement. I don't need my phone or social media and I feel peace.' We worked long-term with the young people to enable them to access opportunities and support.

On a personal level, growing up in a working-class urban town, we didn't have much 'green space', but I can remember the freedom of cycling (quite some distance) to a woodland on the edge of new housing developments. It felt vast and magical and I felt wild and free and usually got home covered in red clay mud and with a treasure trove of stones, acorns, leaves and other exciting finds stuffed in my pocket. It was also an escape from the anger and violence that regularly characterised my household, and perhaps unconsciously taught me at a young age that nature was an ally, a place of safety for me.

Nowadays, I am hugely privileged to live in a beautiful part of the world where I walk every day, and a few years ago I set up allotment plots in my community where we have children, pensioners, families and individuals enjoying the space – my own small plot gives me great joy and challenge! The cyclical and seasonal rhythm of gardening is grounding and nurturing and caring for plants, growing fresh food, physical activity and just 'being' in a beautiful place give me peace, hope, inspiration, creativity and a sense of the sacred which restores and renews me. During lockdown, I set up a seed and plant swap; it was a small thing, but created joy and connection when people found new plants or seeds on their doorsteps or collected them safely from outside someone else's home.

With support and access to opportunities, learning to live well with our mental health struggles can lead to moments of joy and in my experience nature is a gentle, faithful partner in this: as we care for the earth, she cares for us. This is the best medicine for my own mental health and I have seen it help many other people too. Nature truly offers her goodness to all.

Rachel McCann

Notes:

1. *Revelations of Divine Love,* Julian of Norwich

2. *Nature, Biodiversity and Health: An Overview of Interconnections*, World Health Organisation, 2021

3. *www.thrive.org.uk, https://trellisscotland.org.uk*

4. See *Coronavirus: Mental Health in the Pandemic*, Mental Health Foundation

Cocoa the wonder dog

In July 2003, Cocoa the Wonder Dog came into our lives. This was a big step for us (some in the family would say a crazy step), since, being confirmed cat people, we had not really had a relationship with a dog. And, like decisions in many families, this was not a unanimous one.

But it has proven to be a wise choice. For during those long, difficult months of surgery, chemotherapy and hospital stays, which followed our son's diagnosis of Stage 4 cancer, we always had someone at home waiting for us – filled with unconditional love and never-ending hope. I always thought it was true with cats, but Cocoa reminded us that pets are visible signs of that invisible grace God fills us with in each and every moment of our lives.

And Cocoa got us out of the house, especially on those mornings when bed seemed so safe and warm, and on those evenings when all we wanted to do was to veg out in front of the TV. Cats are perfectly content to take care of their business, in their way and time, but dogs – especially a dog like Cocoa – demand to be walked!

And so we did – through puddles; in August heat; shuffling through snow, and trying not to slip on the ice underneath – we walked and walked and walked … And along the way – on starry nights and cloudy days, in times of uncertainty as well as faithfulness, with tears marring our vision and joy bubbling on our lips – God was at work in our lives with the gentle presence of the Holy Spirit, and the healing grace of Jesus Christ.

We have grown accustomed to the belief that healing comes through medication, medical teams, hospitals, wonder treatments. And it does happen that way. But healing also comes in quiet moments: in the gentle hand on a shoulder, in eating a meal prepared by a neighbour, in the prayers of a community of faith, in the silent moments of the night. All too often, however, we are not alert enough to these moments and ways in which the healing power of God is poured upon us.

God does healing work in many remarkable ways, and often through rather 'unremarkable' people, and sometimes, even through a 'dumb animal' like Cocoa.

Note: We had been looking for a dog on and off for months, when we discovered Cocoa. She was the first dog, in all that searching, who approached us, rather than our approaching her first. Not long ago, there was a story on the news about a study which showed that some dogs have a special 'sense' by which they are able to 'smell' cancer in a person. We adopted Cocoa about two months before our son was diagnosed with cancer, and probably at the time when it was 'growing' within him. Gives one pause.

Thom M Shuman

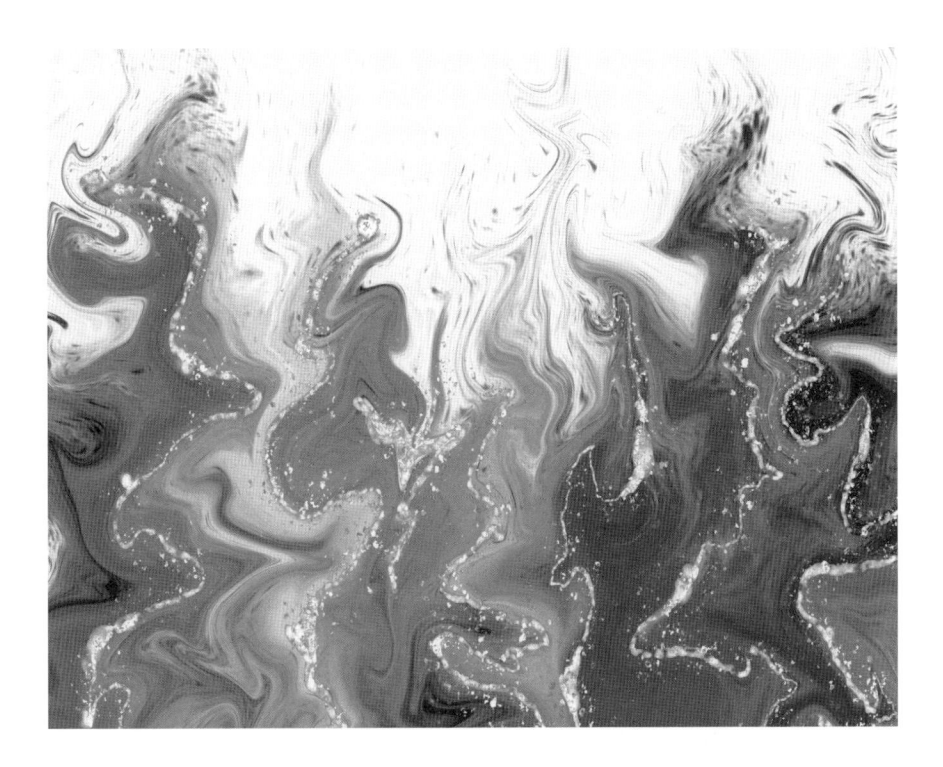

Writing as therapeutic process

As a narrative therapist, I often use writing as a therapeutic tool. For some people it is very helpful to write thoughts and feelings down, as one client once told me: 'I write, and that's the first part of the process. Reading my words then helps me to understand.' I find writing often moves people from a position of 'being stuck' to processing complex thoughts and feelings.

Patrick was an Anglican priest who described himself as 'depressed' and feeling 'angry all the time'. He went on to tell me that: 'Depression stops me feeling. It is a state of non-being. Just dead inside.' He finds talking difficult; writing, however, comes much more naturally to him, and most of our work was through writing and e-mail. Following are some excerpts from his journal, which he kept for over a year and which has been published in full elsewhere.[1]

30th April

Dear Diary,

A story came to me in the night:

Once upon a time there was a young boy. A saint in the making. His face shone with innocence and joy. Everything he touched turned into the colours of the rainbow. Each night, however, when he went home, the light and joy and colour were sucked out of him by a large vampire bat that hung in the corner of his home. It had the face of the Devil. It never moved or spoke, just hung there in brooding silence.

His mother was a very holy woman and tried to keep him joyful. 'Leave him be,' she said of the bat. 'He's not hurting you. He doesn't really exist at all.' Every day she went to the church to say her prayers and collect a bag full of blessings for the boy. So, the boy went about his life and ignored the bat as best he could, his face shining with joy.

The bat travelled with him in his heart, however. It lay alongside the blessings, until one day it spread its wings and said, 'I'm going to devour you.' The boy asked, 'Why? I've always just let you be.' The bat just grinned 'that's my secret' and he ate away the boy's soul, taking all of the joy and the brightness from the boy's world.

I was reading some of the G.K. Chesterton's writing today and came across this line: *'I caught him, with an unseen hook and an invisible line which is long enough to let him wander to the ends of the world, and still to bring him back with a twitch upon the thread'* (from *The Innocence of Father Brown,* 1911).

Although Chesterton was alluding to God twitching the thread – it feels sometimes as if it is something totally evil that twitches me back and that God (if he exists) is powerless to intervene.

7th May

Still having nightmares, and they have spread to waking moments. I suddenly find myself shaking, terrified without reason. Something simple like a glimpse of a face half-known, a smell of perfume, a purple cloth and I can feel my pulse racing. I feel sick and want to run. It happened the other day in the local supermarket. I couldn't go through the till. I had to abandon my trolley halfway down the aisle. Perhaps I am going mad.

Sue asked me if I had ever experienced these kind of feelings when I was a small child, but I haven't. I think that perhaps she thinks there is some kind of 'abuse' in my history, but I really had a very ordinary childhood. My parents were OK – well, my dad used to get depressed, but nothing out of the ordinary. I keep coming back to his face on the day of my ordination though. Not sure why.

18th May

I decided to take the bull by the horns and talk to my parents about my childhood to see if there is anything I should know about. Nothing out of the ordinary – apart from my grandfather dying, which I guess is normal and was not distressing to me. He was after all in his 80s and I had only met him two or three times.

Talking to my dad, however, I realised that he had been more depressed than I realised. I asked him about the tears he shed when I was ordained. He made some lame excuse and changed the subject. That, I thought, was the end of the matter, but a few days later I received a letter from him – I can't ever remember receiving a letter from him, so when I saw his writing on the envelope, I felt quite sick and really anxious.

The letter Patrick received from his father gave an account of how his father had been sexually abused as a young man by his village priest. That letter was the key that helped Patrick to start to understand both his relationship with his parents and his own ambivalence towards the church and faith. Towards the end of our work together Patrick wrote:

> I have written myself into a different place. Along with the Bible, I have been studying the Quran and the Torah, looking at God's interaction with the world, and written long commentaries on how the scripture relates to God's relationship with me. Sue looked a bit glum when I suggested she read it! I can however begin to see a new relationship with God emerging. Before my understandings were based on assumptions that were not true (both about me, my family and the world) and I accept that I will never completely 'know'; they will remain mysteries and that is OK …

Susan Dale

Note:

1. See *The Secret Keepers: Narratives Exploring the Inter- and transgenerational Effects of Childhood Sexual Abuse and Violence*, Susan Dale, Cambridge Scholars Publications, 2013

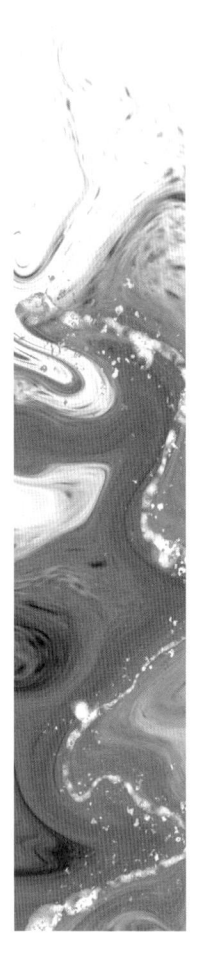

Some things that make me feel better

'Working in the garden'

'Looking at sunlight on a leaf, and planting bulbs for the spring'

'The cat purring in my lap'

'Listening to John Lennon singing "Whatever gets you through the night"'

'Calling up my good friend Jasmine'

'Making love!'

'Community film nights'

'Getting off Facebook for a while'

'Making hot chocolate and taking a nice hot bath.'

'Taking a walk down the rigs'

'Cleaning the house'

'Going shopping'

'Volunteering at the drop-in centre'

'Writing out my soul'

'Playing the piano and being totally in the now.'

'Going somewhere like the North Beach – and screaming'

Various

Community

Our mutual dependence

At the preparation meeting for a visit to Iona, one of the members of the Community Mental Health Chaplaincy Group asked: 'How will our group be described?'

This question expresses one of the common anxieties that surround mental health. It is the experience of many people that once they are diagnosed 'schizophrenic' or 'manic depressive' these become labels.

In 2002, an anti-stigma campaign on mental health in Scotland was launched called 'See me: I'm a person, not a label'. In the chaplaincy, we sought this as a first step for churches and faith communities. We believe that Jesus always saw people rather than labels.

The second step is to recognise that within faith communities there are so many people with so much hidden and locked-up potential. Those who have struggled with mental health problems invariably have a sensitivity and compassion that can contribute creatively to any caring organisation and to society. A member of our group played the guitar in a day centre for children with Down's Syndrome and unlocked some of the shackles of their world. We believe that Jesus brought out potential in people that others never even recognised was there.

Thirdly, we need to recognise our common need for healing. Although the statistics say that one in three of us have mental health problems, all of us have known depression or anxiety or felt despair to some degree and are somewhere on the mental health spectrum.

If we take that to heart, then there is no more 'us' and 'them'. We believe that Jesus challenged us to recognise our mutual dependence.

Iain Whyte, former Community Mental Health Chaplain in Edinburgh

A psalm of hope

A piece which connects access to a healthy diet to good mental health, written on the day (in April 2021) when the Commons Environment, Food and Rural Affairs All-Party Committee called for a law enshrining 'a right to food', having found that more than 7 million people in the UK live in food poverty ...

Why the exponential increase in need;
why have charitable responses become the norm?
The voices of people living in poverty
cry out in distress.
Despite their cries, a shameful currency of vouchers,
donated foods and dateline surplus
rolls on and on.

Supermarket collection points
groan with donations
as a pandemic exacerbates and escalates a chronic crisis.
Here in the UK, the well-being of hungry children
hangs in the balance,
until someone with the cachet to speak out on their behalf
humiliates the decision-makers.
We know the health impacts of poverty will be a long, slow burn.
We know the outcomes, when processed foods become staples
and 5-a-day becomes an unaffordable luxury.
We know deprivation decimates development
and shatters the life chances of hungry children
and the mental health of adults.
We know the 'right to food' is a basic human right.

What have we learned in the twenty years as the foodbank culture grew to become an epidemic?

How long will 20% of the population remain
trapped by systemic failure?

How long till the voices of lived experience shape
what actually happens locally?

What's it really like to grow up dependent on free school meals?

Are community leaders proactively assessing volunteer roles
to create training and employment?

How are statutory, charitable and commercial sectors connecting
local resources to establish dignified, sustainable solutions to need?

How are foodbanks accountable within local communities
for their role in distributing donations?

Where are the prophetic voices challenging this escalating injustice?

In frustration and anger, I wonder, have I become part of the problem?
The all-consuming operation:
collecting, sorting, weighing, storing and recording.
Repacking, redistributing and administering provisions,
an energy-sapping process which distorts perspectives.

However well-intentioned, local communities are caught up
in an ever-increasing 'hamster-wheel' with no clear exit strategy,
inadvertently perpetuating a subsistence-level existence
which traps their poverty-stricken neighbours.

Creator of the earth,
open our eyes to the hope of your love all around.
The promise for new growth in the garden,
the verge, car park and churchyard.
Place where communities can come together
to dig, sow, tend and grow.
Places for harvesting and sharing the joy of abundance
as seasons unfold.
The peeling and chopping,
creating time for relationships to emerge
while food is prepared.
The kneading and shaping
opening opportunities for cultures and stories to be shared
and understood.

How we long for the dignity of living together
with an abundance of difference and potential,
all people equally and wonderfully made in the image of God.

Christine Jones

Cyrenians: On supporting emotional and mental well-being during the pandemic and beyond

'At Cyrenians we tackle the causes and consequences of homelessness. We understand that there are many routes into homelessness, and that there is no "one size fits all" approach to supporting people towards more positive and stable futures. That's why all our work is values-led and relationships-based. We meet people where they are, and support them towards where they want to be ...'

From the Cyrenians website (https://cyrenians.scot)

Many of the people we journey with at Cyrenians have experienced trauma which shapes the way they experience the world. It has often limited their ability to make the best of who they are, taking them into behaviours and choices which often exacerbate the impact of their trauma. This has a huge effect on their mental and emotional well-being.

We are not, nor do we have the ambition to be, clinicians. We do not offer therapy or medical solutions. What we bring is the time, capacity and willingness to be in relationship with those we support. We take a person-centred approach which places the individual at the heart of any solutions; they define success, not us. In building trusted relationships, those we support experience being cared for, not being let down, judged or rejected when they stumble or act out the consequences of their trauma in negative behaviours. Our approach uses Roger's *'unconditional positive regard'* – whatever the person's story, their past actions or decisions, we simply see them now, in front of us, as them: as a person with potential and hope.

In this last year, creating these kinds of professional, but personal, deeply human, trusted relationships has been hugely challenging. Presence is crucial in making them work, in nurturing them from very small steps and apparently false starts. The chances of them breaking down were significant. And the impact on people's emotional well-being was profound. When relationships are tough anyway, to have your ability to be in relationship limited by lockdown was extremely difficult for the folk we support, tipping many into a return to harmful behaviours again.

We did a huge amount digitally. Where it was needed we provided both equipment and Wi-Fi, and when required, training and support. We worked hard at getting folk used to working in digital spaces, to talking on the phone and on video calls and using Chat and messaging. It had some unexpected outcomes. Our recovery group, initially sceptical and limited in capacity, discovered they could access recovery groups all over the world at any time of the day and night. Suddenly they were sharing their stories with people in Los Angeles and Melbourne and in many places in between.

We rediscovered the power of the written word. Staff and volunteers wrote hundreds of letters and cards to the folk we support. The feedback was really positive. It was something about the personal touch, that someone cared enough to sit and handwrite something to them.

We held online ceilidhs – people jigging away in their front rooms. And we did lots and lots of garden and doorstep conversations, at times in awful weather. Digital is good, but physical presence is, in the end, irreplaceable for feeding our inner well-being.

We also supported over 100 families in conflict, using digital spaces to enable them to have the conversations they needed with each other. The pain of being in conflict whilst unable to leave the family home had a devastating effect on the emotional well-being of many parents and their children. We found many, though not all, young people fed back that they were able to say more in the digital space than they might have face to face. It's not just because young people are 'digital natives': there's something freeing about having a little distance when being vulnerable with an adult, even one they trust, such as the Cyrenians' staff member supporting them. It is an insight we will take into our post-pandemic thinking, ensuring we continue offering ways of supporting people that work for them.

We used our outdoor spaces, our farm, community gardens and food depot to create new opportunities for young people who were already struggling at school, with the transition to online learning leaving them further away from their peers: small groups of 15- and 16-year-olds getting out, doing physical work, learning about the power of collaboration and their emotional well-being fed by the power of connection. The vast majority discovered in themselves the courage and capacity to apply for college, and were successful, something unthinkable at the start of the pandemic.

Although we adapted and reconfigured the whole organisation's activity, we never lost sight of our core principle of taking a holistic approach:

always seeking ways to support the whole person and not just focusing on the 'presenting issue'. Throughout the pandemic we kept doing whatever we could to maintain the trusted relationships which are the bedrock of what we do; allowing us to create the space to discover the right solutions for each individual and then empowering them to make those happen. We know that healthy relationships are also the bedrock of good emotional well-being. We knew if we kept the relationships going, we would be providing the best possible support at a time when literally everyone, us included, was finding it a struggle.

Ewan Aitken, CEO of Cyrenians

https://cyrenians.scot/real-stories

A man has died

A man has died. A young man. A man aged 20. A man in hotel detention. A man in McLays Guest House. A man formerly housed by Mears Group Ltd. A man. A man given a name of Adnan Olbeh. The news of this saddest of tragedies is buzzing on my phone with incongruously cheery ring tones. I change the tone.

The waves of incredulity have been circulating among the ragged, fiercely organised and indefatigably creative network of activists and workers who have committed themselves to working with and for refugees. Positive Action, Unity, the Night Shelter, Ubuntu, the Scottish Refugee Council, Maryhill Integration Network, No Evictions, Refuweegee – the list is long, is civic.

The love and tensions, solidarities and differences are vital to the work of enduring alongside those who suffer the systematic cruelties of the UK's Home Office policies towards refugees and asylum seekers. These cruelties are carefully constructed. They involve regular court cases which find the Home Office to have broken the law; they involve years of appeals and the most mind-numbingly tenacious work by immigration lawyers and case workers.

A man has died. A man with friends. Family. A man from Syria. A man seeking refuge. A man.

A man has died.

This happened in Glasgow when protest is difficult and gatherings cannot take place, because we need to protect one another, to shield, to make many, many sanctuaries.

Nor can we gather in our usual meetings and committees or verify easily the reports from the asylum seekers reaching us via those affected, that they were given half an hour to leave their flats; rounded up into vans and decanted unceremoniously into hotels in the city where they were to share food and accommodation; their utterly pitiful asylum support of £37.50 a week was stopped; and they were full of fear. People seeking asylum. Here. And they are full of fear. Here. Here. And during Ramadan. Those who do the lion's share of the real work of hosting and helping are the New Scots in Glasgow; the ethnic minorities; the people who can speak the mother languages of those who are so, so afraid.

It's hard to understand what we say in English at the best of times, in this city of Glasgow, but even harder when you are afraid. Your brain freezes; your words stumble. My friends doing this work tell me that they speak – at a two-metre distance, of course, of course, always compliant – to men weeping on the park benches of the city, who have been turned out of individual flats by Mears and are now sharing in hotels. And they are so afraid. Mears, Serco, the Home Office. Names on our lips which we speak with shame.

Refuweegee have delivered 5000 packages of care so far. And they would be the first to underscore that they are not the only ones in the city doing food and medicine runs.

Underneath this figure are all the families of New Scots in the city dropping off parcels of *injera* and *ghaat* and *berbera* on the doorsteps of those with newborns; those who are ill; those who are working our deliveries; cleaning our hospitals.

And awaiting the fall of the next sword of Damocles from the Home Secretary's hand. When I do this work, the police don't stop me or question me. When the New Scots do this, they are followed home, doubted. It's just how it is. It's not how it should be.

A man has died. In amongst the horror of the UK's dreadful, dreadful death toll – a death toll which is the pure face of policies of greed and carelessness – is the death of this man. Far from home. He had asked us for help. The detention systems writ large across our cities separate you. They inculcate fear. They shrink to next to nothing the circles of love and care around you.

Our time of confinement, for the keeping safe of one another, is not 'lockdown'. The years of living in asylum systems are 'lockdown'.

The world has changed. We don't need to look any further than the saddest loss of a young life, of Adnan Olbeh, to see exactly how the Home Office is already treating those seeking refuge now.

And given that we know that the treatment of those seeking refuge works as a test ground for how we might treat those in rent arrears; those with disabilities; with mental health struggles; those who can't work easily; those whose visas are insecure; those who can't afford nannies or cleaners; those who will lose their jobs in the great recession that has also come upon us; then we know, again, how it is – not how it will be, but how it is, already.

The meetings have happened, despite it all. The city, her activists, her politicians and the Scottish MPs have been clear and like terriers on the trouser leg of the Prime Minister and Home Secretary.

David Linden MP using his question at Prime Minister's Questions to press on the accommodation crisis; Councillor Jen Layden has written to the Home Secretary; there are five very clear demands from the Scottish Refugee Council.

We want answers – yes – from a Home Office and Home Secretary who have more than 15 years worth of reports and evidence on the dangers and lethal consequences of their policies of hostility.

The refugee background experts, activists, academics and NGOs have done their work, written their reports, presented their evidence – and all that has happened is further hostility.

No respecters of evidence, or experts, our Home Office.

A man has died. The world changed and the hostility was ramped up to protect the profits of the rich, by increasing the suffering of the most vulnerable amongst us. And to every one single person who says 'we must look after our own': even if you cannot strip those poisoned words from your tongue, you must know, must know by now, that we are – and always were – connected by webs of microbes in the very air we breathe; that your health is my health; and that what is coming to visit you in your terrified speech is what has visited those who have sought help amongst us. You must know that when you need help yourself that the words which pronounce a death sentence are the very words you are speaking.

A man has died. A man asked us for help. To be amongst us. Alive.

We took an hour to join so many in online vigil in mourning the loss of this young Syrian man. Some walked by the guest house and laid flowers. The proprietors binned them. Flowers, it seems, are too unmasking, too potent a symbol, too clear a sign.

Every life lost to the asylum system – a system predicated on cruelty and injustice – is preventable. But for now – now – silence.

The surge of angry tears;
the waste of it all.
The cruelty.
The sheer hopelessness;
the unutterable loneliness.
The knowing of it in our own intimate lives.
The not knowing of it.
And in our gathered silence –
strewn with the images
of cardboard signs
and wilting garden flowers – is our love,
the resolute love for humanity
and international solidarity
that beats high and hard
against the great breast bone of this city, still.
Rest in Peace,
friend I never met.
Rest in Peace.

Alison Phipps, 2020

'Research suggests that asylum seekers are five times more likely to have mental health needs than the general population … However, data shows that they are less likely to receive support than the general population.'

From the Mental Health Foundation website (www.mentalhealth.org.uk)

Musical hospitality, music-making and mental health

In 1997 I went to Iona to work for the Iona Community, a time which became the start of my musical journey (as much as a spiritual one), in particular, learning to enable music with others. Knowing that I was to be resident there for quite some time, I had brought a small *djembe* with me with the hope that I would learn how to play it on my time off – preferably on a remote beach out of public earshot! Within a couple of months, I was playing several times a week; not to the gentle accompaniment of waves and seagulls, but right in the heart of worship in a medieval abbey.

Why? Ultimately it was a lot to do with hospitality – in music and in worship. Unlike a regular church congregation, the assembled worshippers in the Abbey would be vastly different at every service, due to the majority of the congregation being made up of island visitors. Each evening, the congregation could consist of people from any denomination or level of church involvement – including those with no Christian experience or belief at all. This meant that we could take nothing for granted as far as a 'canon' of hymnody was concerned – a hackneyed old favourite for some of us could be entirely unknown to others.

Potentially, there's nothing more exclusive than everyone else knowing the song that you don't – reaffirming your status as an 'outsider'. In Iona, the intent of worship was to be a place where God's welcome was extended to everyone. This meant that if we were to practise a 'musical hospitality', then we had to offer a place for everyone within our music, rather than simply do music to, or for, them.

Practically, this meant including simple, achievable songs, often taking a few minutes to teach them before the service, so that by the time they came round in worship, they would be familiar. A number of the songs were from parts of the wider world church – Africa, Latin America, India. I could see first-hand how these songs were able to involve a much broader spectrum of people, as they did not rely on reading music or words, and the cyclical structure enabled them to be quickly learned. This became most apparent in a week where members of the L'Arche Community (involving adults with additional support needs) were staying in one of the island Centres, and a group of theologians in the other. It was one of these magic Iona weeks where people from vastly different backgrounds are brought unexpectedly together. During worship I could see the participants from L'Arche mostly listening to the longer hymns – yet when the shorter, world church songs were sung, they were able to join in with gusto, and participate on an equal basis – and more confidently than some of the theologians!

The entire experience of Iona-style musical hospitality stayed with me long after I had moved back to the mainland, and ultimately forged my subsequent career path. Nowadays I work making music together with a variety of different groups: from people in intensive psychiatric care, to adults and children with additional support needs, people with dementia, and refugees – all of whom speak the common language of music, and particularly rhythm.

Contrary to what many people believe (barely a workshop passes without someone explaining that 'I've got no rhythm'), no previous experience is necessary in order to participate in the creation of successful music together – there's something about the structure of rhythmic music which enables people to join in across vastly differing levels of ability. It's not just for the 'musical' or 'talented' – it's for everyone, and can offer powerful experiences of inclusion and participation, particularly for people who, for one reason or another, are often excluded from musical activity. It also depends on (and nurtures) skills such as listening, communication, self-control, self-expression and group responsibility.

These capacities of communicative and cooperative musicality have deep roots not only in the way we first learn to share time and space with another person, but deep within our human evolutionary process. In our own lives, acts of dialogue, turn-taking, listening, aligning and responding are found in our earliest interactions with our caregivers – and are the same skills we use in making music with others. Cambridge-based professor of music and science, Ian Cross, makes a convincing case for the role of shared musicality in human evolution – where the *'floating intentionality'* (i.e. non-specificity) of group music-making could act as a behavioural rehearsal for a group.[1] The act of playing music around the campfire could offer a relatively inconsequential space for engaging in acts of cooperation, coordination and social bonding – so that in situations when it mattered (such as hunting the mammoth), the group would function more successfully than the tribe in the next valley that didn't sing, dance and make music together.

These potentialities of music are still very much in evidence today – many corporations have used drumming as a tool to bring their teams together, working musically in the 'inconsequential' space in order to bring their freshly honed skills to the workplace. And in mental health, it offers an open door to community and group interaction for those who may struggle with it. Being together in music means that it's perfectly possible to be part of a group without having to talk about yourself, or come up with the right answers; to gently build relationships through music, so that when the opportunity comes for actual conversation, the barriers have been lowered, just a little – but perhaps enough to stay and talk.

I've had the opportunity to see the long-term consequences of this, in the 15-year relationship with the drumming group The Buddy Beat,[2] based in Paisley, just outside Glasgow. Originally growing from a project started in the NHS, the idea behind it was to offer a transitional space from an activity people could experience while in hospital – to one that offers social inclusion within the wider community. Today we have around 20-30 members, some who have been part of the group since its beginning. What has happened is that, over the years, genuine community has formed. Through drumming together, members – nearly all of whom suffered profoundly from social isolation – built relationships with each other. Deep, meaningful relationships. Members check in on each other, have formed clubs and businesses together – and credit the group and each other with keeping them well and out of hospital.

It feels like things have come full circle – thanks to those initial experiences on Iona. Learning to practise a musical hospitality congruent with a theology of welcome – where all have a place at the table, every voice counts, and each person has a unique gift within the music of a community. To extend a welcome to people who dance to a different beat.

Jane Bentley

Notes:

1. See, for example, 'Music and communication in music psychology', Ian Cross, Sage Journals, 2014

2. www.thebuddybeat.org

The Buddy Beat

My own mental health declined in 2006 and by 2008 I was a lost soul. I knew something had to change, having considered myself at the end of the line. Out of the blue I had an unexpected drumming experience with Dr Jane Bentley, who invited me along to the Buddy Beat. I instantly found that the music let me leave my worries at the door, giving me the first peace in many years. I kept attending, and as the weeks turned into months, then into years, I found that the things lost to me – self-confidence, self-worth, friendship – were returning bit by bit. After a while I was asked at an event how I had found being part of the group, and I replied: 'It's the one place where I can be me.' The Buddy Beat saved my life in no short measure, and also opened it outwards, giving me the empowerment of performance, giving me back my creativity and leading me into volunteering and employment.

I am not the only person to benefit of course, and I'd like to share another couple of examples from the group. Derek had been out of work for some time, and joined Buddy Beat despite never having been a part of any community group, wanting something to give him that life spark we all look for. He enjoyed the structure and sense of belonging, and found his own well-being improved. Derek succeeded in gaining employment as a peer support worker in our local mental health hospital and has now moved on to full-time work at our local general hospital.

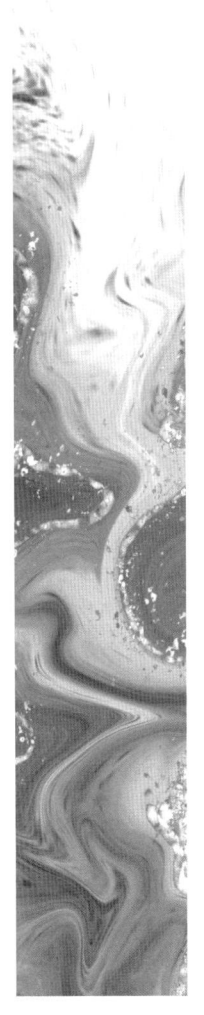

Stacey also needed an activity to improve her self-isolation and confidence. She saw Buddy Beat perform in public in 2014 and was inspired to give it a go, and has blossomed since then: becoming an integral part of our membership. Using our group as a launch pad, Stacey has volunteered with ROAR, a local older adults' organisation, and Flexi-Care, who provide clubs for young people within the Autism/Asperger's spectrum, and has received an award for her work at their recent annual awards bash! She has also joined a mental health drama group. We all see the change in her and appreciate that she can still find time to join us each week.

I firmly believe that the best way to move forward is to not let your mental health hold you back. There is a lot out there and with a little luck you can find it and reap the benefit.

Tom Chalmers, the Buddy Beat

Pastoral conversation recollected

She sat with me for about two hours and talked nearly non-stop. She told me she was being persecuted and bullied by those around her. Her family rejected her. That her parents loved her sisters much more than they loved her. How she knew things about people that they wouldn't want her to tell. How her sister's husband had made a pass at her and how she wanted to tell her sister but couldn't. How her neighbour in the upstairs flat was persecuting her by stamping heavily across the ceiling of the room when she tried to sleep at night. How she was scared every time she opened the door of her flat that she would meet her upstairs neighbour. How that neighbour always looked at her in a funny way …

And on and on …

I listened.

I nodded and made a few interjections, but mostly I just let her talk.

Talking is good for you – so they say.

And though I doubt that much of what she said was true, it was all real enough to her to be a powerful and damaging influence on her life.

The doctors gave her pills.

John Butterfield

The Asclepion of Pergamon

The Asclepion of Pergamon, in present-day Turkey, is credited with being the world's first ever psychiatric hospital. It was a temple complex dedicated, as its name indicates, to Asclepius, the Greek god of medicine, and was a major centre of healing in the ancient world between the 4th century BC and the 2nd century AD.

Although belonging to an ancient world and culture very different from our own, some of the methods and treatments used in the Asclepion in the treatment of mental illness bear a striking resemblance to some of those in use today.

From the start of treatment patients were encouraged to relax; there was a library and theatre on site. After a while settling in, patients were invited to sleep in cubicles along the side of the 'sacred way', an underground tunnel which connected the outer complex with the inner worship area. In the morning they would ascend a few steps into the light of the temple, symbolising their journey through the darkness of illness into the light of healing.

The next step was to devise the treatment plan. It was believed that the god would come to them in their dreams, and the temple priests would help to interpret what the god had revealed. The best and most effective treatment comes when patient and therapist work together! Treatments on offer included music therapy, massage, exercise, talking therapies and medication.

The important thing for us to note is that here, psychiatric therapy was offered at a place of worship and in the context of worship. Are our places of worship also places of healing? One local church once placed a poster outside its doors which read *'This Church is a health centre'*. Could you say that about your church?

Gill Dascombe

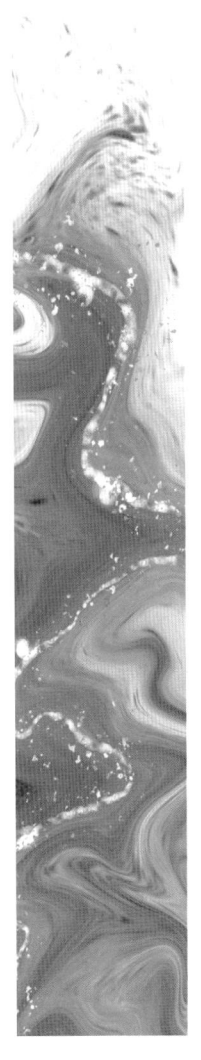

Fellowship at the State Hospital

For over 52 years, Iona Community associate and musician Philip Fox has been regularly volunteering at the State Hospital in Carstairs in South Lanarkshire, Scotland.

'I was sick and you took care of me, I was in prison and you visited me.'
Matthew 25:36 (NRSV)[1]

I remember, as a teenager and a newly committed Christian, being disturbed by the challenge of this verse. Only when I moved to Scotland, however, did the opportunity arise to actively respond to it.

In 1970 I was able to join a small group of volunteers visiting men, and at that time women, held in Carstairs State Hospital, which in those days had an east and west wing separated by the main railway line. Our visits were fortnightly to a specified ward, changed every 6 months or so, and we spent our time in conversation and 'news-sharing' of happenings from outside. In those days access to external news was more limited, just as effective treatment regimes were less available. The sad sight of patients sitting in a 'vegetative state' with mouth twitching (tardive dyskinesia) under haloperidol drug control was all too common.

Suppressing uncontrolled physical and mental activity often added to the difficulties of communication.

Much time was given over to listening, becoming aware of some of the tragic circumstances, often family-related, contributing to why people were there. For some a sense of worthlessness and rejection could not be hidden, particularly when family connections were severed and visiting was non-existent. In the circumstances, awareness of our helplessness to do little more than listen had a particularly telling effect.

But I realised that weakness could open us to the Very Being, the Spirit of God within us, able to help and transform all lives (including my own) when problems/issues are identified and acknowledged.

Thus a sense of purpose in what we as volunteers were doing quickly became apparent: in us – a sense of warmth, joy and value confirmed the good use of whatever talents we individually could use there; in the patients – visible changes in attitudes, positive focus on the Gospel, with an emerging awareness and development of their own gifts/talents in rebuilding broken lives.

In 1970 Rayne was one such patient, seemingly a poet. I thought I would 'help out' by buying a copy of his first book of poetry, *The Spark of Joy*, just then published. During subsequent visits I also copied in blank spaces of my book his latest 'creations'.

Imagine then my amazement and humbling to read, in 2002, in the *Glasgow Herald*, an obituary of Rayne Mackinnon: the international award-winning poet.

The following, entitled 'Stillness', is one of his:

> *The ward seems made for peace today. Like specks*
> *Of dust in the sun's rays, men's voices drift*
> *Along the corridor. Then, the soft smack*
> *Of dominoes upon a table. Doors*
> *Bang timidly, afraid to break the calm;*
> *Even the jovial wireless seems subdued.*
> *For all inside, it seems, have taken note*
> *Of a perfect day. Shouldering aside*
> *The stubborn haze, the hills have lost their shame.*
> *The bare blue sky thrusts back small straggling clouds*
> *Into the distance and oblivion.*
> *The soil, unburdened, opens all its pores,*
> *Sucks in the stillness of the air. This mood*
> *Will vanish soon, no doubt, but now the whole*
> *Rough world seems held, and cradled in the calm.*[2]

Unwittingly Rayne raised my awareness of how God-given talents can surely shine in seemingly unlikely places! Much has changed since the '70s but that potential remains, not only as a factor motivating my continuing involvement today, but by being progressively inbuilt in the way the hospital runs.

Carstairs, in combination with the Scottish Prison Service, is now undoubtedly a 'flagship' for the NHS, providing a second-to-none environment where mentally and physically disturbed men have opportunities to show their hidden potentials for good. The facilities now available reflect unprecedented care, education (witnessed in the recently instituted internal Awards Ceremony events) and treatment, which includes a stated recognition of the benefits of spiritual input.

So the weekly Christian Fellowship Meetings play a significant role, alongside ecumenical services taken by the appointed Chaplains, at which I generally provide the music. Indeed the importance of music-making can hardly be overstressed. Over the last 30 years or so teaching and singing new songs and hymns has provided a wonderful expression for the lads.

A typical meeting commences with a rapid-fire of perhaps a dozen *Mission Praise* items chosen by them, and an opportunity to teach some new ones. There has even been an occasion to write a hymn specially for them.

We share and reflect on a Gospel reading, before concluding with a time of prayer. The men also have access to Bible-reading notes, which I use from time to time as a basis for our fellowship meetings.

It has been a lasting joy and privilege for me over more than 52 years to be given the opportunity to use what God-given aptitudes and talents I have to help open doors for others at Carstairs, trying to meet the original challenge confronting me as a teenager.

All praise be to our Creator.

Philip Fox

Notes:

1. Passages from NRSV copyright 1989, Division of Christian Education of the National Council of the Churches of Christ in the United States of America. Used by permission. All rights reserved.

2. 'Stillness', by Rayne Mackinnon, from *The Spark of Joy*, Caithness Books, 1970.

    I have tried my best to discover the copyright holder of Rayne Mackinnon's poetry but have not been successful. I have included the poem because I think it is important that his voice is heard. (Ed.)

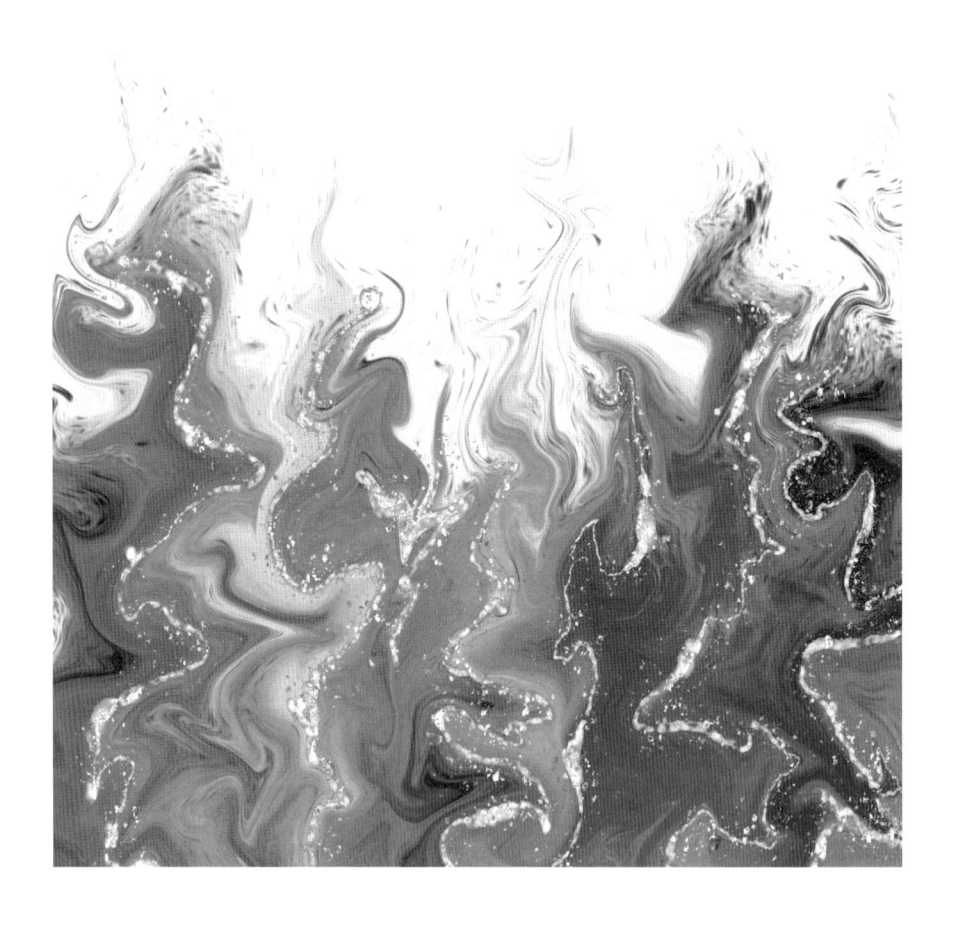

About the authors

Ewan Aitken is a member of the Iona Community, and also CEO of Cyrenians, a charity committed to tackling the causes and consequences of homelessness.

Warren Bardsley is a retired Methodist minister living in Lichfield. He is a member of the Iona Community and its Common Concern Network for Palestine. He is involved in the local City of Sanctuary movement, interested in music (of most kinds) and passionate about the game of cricket.

Elizabeth Baxter continues her therapeutic, liturgical and theological ministry at Holy Rood House in Thirsk. As a priest, she enjoys accompanying people on their spiritual journey. Being an edge-walker herself, Elizabeth enjoys spending time 'on the borders', walking along the edge of Spittal beach with family and friends and her dog, Rafi.

Jane Bentley has been associated with the Iona Community for twenty-five years, first volunteering in the Community's shop. She works as a musician in health and social care settings, and firmly believes everyone has the capacity for musical well-being.

Patrick Bentley is a volunteer therapist with Freedom from Torture. He previously worked as a social worker with Children's Services and in the NHS as a Child and Adolescent Mental Health therapist and a manager.

Ruth Burgess: 'I live in Dunblane. I enjoy wandering around my garden, reading, writing and editing. When I get a chance I delight in paddling along the seashore, though getting my socks back on isn't getting any easier.'

John Butterfield recently retired after a pastoral ministry of 34 years. He has been alongside church members, friends, colleagues and relatives struggling with their mental health and well-being.

Tom Chalmers: 'I am a mental health survivor who now lives a rich life through drumming. I am a workshop facilitator, singer/songwriter (see Rhythm to a T Chalmers on YouTube), creative writer and unofficial support worker too.'

Alex Clare-Young is a pioneer minister in the United Reformed Church and an Iona Community member. Alex writes and speaks regularly on LGBTQ+ identities, neurodiversity and theology.

Luke Concannon has early memories of listening to live music, dancing, singing, and putting on plays at his Irish family's parties in Warwickshire. He's been making music in community ever since. Aged 26 he topped the UK and Irish charts with his duo Nizlopi's 'The JCB Song' about singing with has dad after school in the family digger; the band were totally independent, turning down offers from major labels in order to stay true to their ethic of being community-based. The band split in 2009 due to the pressures of holding their ideals together, and Luke has been finding a way back to wholeness since. His 2021 album *Ecstatic Bird in the Burning* saw Luke enter the US and UK folk charts at Number 12 and receive rave reviews: https://lukeconcannon.com

Kathy Crawford is a former foster parent and kinship carer. Many years of experience have shown her how negative childhood experiences, as well as learning difficulties such as ADHD, autism and dyslexia, can all impact on a person's mental health and self-esteem. Kathy admits that she is still learning and, although she may never manage to fully understand the pain and frustration these things cause, she continues to do her best to be supportive.

Tricia Creamer is a member of Poole Methodists, and since 2006 ran a weekly Celtic Colours Group exploring Christian spirituality through Celtic art. She loves writing, teaching the piano and is an associate member of the Iona Community.

Susan Dale is a psychotherapist, author and member of the Iona Community. She currently works for the UHI Inverness within the Wellbeing Team.

Gill Dascombe is a former Vice-President of the Methodist Conference. A retired NHS mental health pharmacist, she is a lay preacher, retreat leader and grandmother of two, living in Bolton.

Christine Dowling has worked predominantly with adults with mental health issues for over 15 years. They have taught her to observe and appreciate life in different ways. Her mum towards the end of her life developed vascular dementia. She forgot the things she enjoyed but then rediscovered them.

About the authors 241

Philip Fox: Influenced by my English 'Methodist' parents became a committed Christian as a teenager, and inheriting father's passion and talents as organist/choirmaster applied them as conductor of a choral union for 43 years. As an associate of the Iona Community, privileged to enjoy spells as Iona Abbey musician and to produce hymns/songs for Wild Goose Publications.

Katie Frost lives in Nottinghamshire and is in her twenties. She is the very proud owner of a young Labrador called Shadow, who brings joy and light to every life he touches.

Laura Gisbourne is a member of the Iona Community Young Adults Group. She lives in Yorkshire with her fiancé and son.

Linda Hill is (almost) retired, having spent most of the last 45 years working with a wide variety of people and a wide variety of the issues that impact our mental health. The gift of that work has been to meet some extraordinary people and to experience the privilege of witnessing their courage and resilience.

Jean Hudson: 'The gift for writing came as a wonderful surprise when I could no longer preach, and had, in quaint Methodist terms, 'sat down' (retired). God's world and God's word continue to provide all the inspiration I could ask for, as well as light in the darkness of recurring depression, to fill the space there always is for hope.'

Peter Charles Jackson is a retired journalist, editor and corporate communications consultant. He's the author of five books of Christian drama sketches, a member of High Weald Poets and an occasional preacher at his parish church in Crowborough, East Sussex.

Ann Jepson: 'I am a retired Anglican priest living in Lancashire and helping out in my local rural parish. I enjoy gardening and travelling and a ministry of spiritual direction and supervision.'

Christine Jones is a wife, mother and Methodist minister who is passionate about food justice.

Thea Joshi works in communications for a mental health charity. She is fiercely passionate about churches becoming safe spaces for anyone living with a mental health problem, and blogs about faith and OCD. She lives in Nottingham and loves tea, dogs and the facepalm emoji.

Janet Lees, a former school chaplain, is a writer and a member of the Lay Community of St Benedict. She enjoys walking and in 2019 she walked from Land's End to John o'Groats. She has an elderly campervan called Bambi and blogs at: https://foowr.org.uk/notesfrombambi. You can follow her on Twitter @Bambigoesforth.

Emma Major is a pioneer lay minister, blind wheelchair user, artist and poet. She has written seven poetry books on disability, grief, mental health, faith and climate change. You can find Emma online at LLMCalling.com or on social media @emmuk74 where she shares her creativity to encourage, bless and affirm people.

Rachel McCann is a former youth, community and social worker who retrained in gardening. Amongst other things, she enjoys her allotment, crafting, foraging, pottery and making soap. She is an associate member of the Iona Community and a published poet and writer, whose work has appeared in a number of books and magazines.

Alastair McIntosh is a founding board member of the GalGael Trust (www.galgael.org) and an Isle of Lewis-raised writer, broadcaster and campaigner: www.alastairmcintosh.com

Rosie Miles is a poet and trainee professional gardener. She formerly taught English within academia, but is now running her own freelance poetry courses and retreats. Rosie lives in Birmingham.

Yvonne Morland has been a member of the Iona Community for 20 years and has contributed writing to many Wild Goose Publications. For more than this period, she has experienced episodes of mental ill health.

David Norman is an associate member of the Iona Community.

Katy Owen: Member of the Iona Community since 1982 and still appreciating the support and challenge of the members.

Susan Palmer has loved and served Jesus with all her heart and soul since she was 11 years old. She is a member of South Street Baptist Church in Exeter.

Neil Paynter is an editor, writer and late-night piano player. Previously he worked in homeless shelters and nursing homes, and picking fruit and as a hospital cleaner.

Alison Phipps is a member of the Iona Community and UNESCO Chair for Refugee Integration through Languages and Arts.

Rosemary Power is a member of the Iona Community and a writer who has been engaged in church and similar work for many years. In recent times she has volunteered with refugees.

Katherine Rennie is a member of the Iona Community and Local Preacher with the Methodist Church. She is a retired family solicitor and mediator.

Bev Robertson: 'Priest, poet and painter, and wildlife sculptor, living and working in Worcestershire. My love of creation and the interconnectedness of life inspires me to write, paint and sculpt to express and focus on the miraculous beauty we inhabit and are called to care for.'

The Rev'd Sr Sandra Sears, CSBC, is a Local Priest in the Anglican Diocese of Willochra in rural South Australia, and a member of the Community of Sts Barnabas and Cecilia. As well as poetry, stories and liturgical resources, she is a composer of songs and hymns suitable for congregational use, especially those in country areas with minimal musical resources.

Robert Shooter: 'I was born in Worksop, North Nottinghamshire. I did a degree in Economics in London and then a post-grad Social Work qualification at Nottingham University, where I met my wife. Our four children, grown-up, are scattered around Britain. Later in life I became ordained and got a degree in Theology and worked as a hospital chaplain. I have an MA in Writing Studies from Edge Hill University, which was so enjoyable, but have always dabbled in creating writing. I also love walking, music and being with our kids, and theirs.'

Thom M Shuman is an associate member of the Iona Community, living in Columbus, Ohio. He is a poet, pastor, lover of words, a struggler and straggler trying to follow Jesus.

Neil Squires is the Chief Executive of Harmeny Education Trust and a member of the Iona Community.

Jan Sutch Pickard: For nearly six years Jan was part of the Iona Community's team working at and welcoming guests to the Abbey and MacLeod Centre, from whom she learned about the stresses under which many live, and the creative moments that can liberate us.

Kathy Swaar: A writer, blogger, retired pastor and teacher, Kathy is the author of *Fine Lines: Walking the Labyrinth of Grief and Loss*. CEO of her family's farm corporation, she oversees the management of their Midwestern US grain farm. When not writing or tending farm business, she can be found reading, watching sports and cooking shows, digging up dead relatives, sewing and collecting cookbooks and antique glassware.

Simon Taylor is the Free Church Chaplain at the University of Exeter and a Baptist minister. He also ministers at South Street Baptist Church, which seeks to offer a welcome and support to those with mental health difficulties. For his own well-being, he walks on Dartmoor and bakes bread to share with others.

Pamela Turner: 'Glasgow-born, I trained for the ministry in Edinburgh and was ordained by the Presbyterian Church of Wales in 1978. After ministry in Wales and Shropshire till 2003 I worked as a healthcare chaplain in Birmingham both in the acute and the mental health sectors. An associate member of the Iona Community and now retired, I am returning to Scotland where I will be spending more time writing.'

Jessica Wachter is a church planter/redeveloper in the Episcopal Church, a wife to Ray, and a cat-mom to Luna. She lives in central Missouri and loves hiking, reading, writing and meeting Jesus on park benches and in laundromats.

Iain Whyte is retired Church of Scotland minister who has been a youth worker in Ghana, a parish minister, a University Chaplain and Head of Christian Aid Scotland. When writing on slavery and racial issues he was a part-time Community Mental Health Chaplain, where he learnt much from those he met. He is an activist on African issues, refugees, food poverty and Palestine, and has been a member of the Iona Community for 56 years.

Rev. Prof. Stephen G Wright is a poet and author, and spiritual director for the Sacred Space Foundation (www.sacredspace.org.uk) and founder of the Kentigern School of Contemplatives (www.kentigern.org.uk). His most recent works are *Heartfullness* and *Burnout: A Spiritual Crisis on the Way Home* (www.sacredspace.org.uk). He is a member of the Iona Community and Hon. Fellow of the University of Cumbria.

Source and acknowledgements

'Alyas' prayer' – by Alyas, from *Standing on Our Stories: The Justice, Peace and Wholeness Commitment of the Iona Community*, Susan Dale, Wild Goose Publications, 2020

'Thank you for old friends' – by Neil Paynter, from *Friends & Enemies: A Book of Short Prayers and Some Ways to Write Your Own*, Ruth Burgess (Ed.), Wild Goose Publications, 2004

'A psalm of thanksgiving', 'A blessing for those who are depressed' and 'A blessing for those who have no one left to talk to' – by Neil Paynter, from *A Book of Blessings: And How to Write Your Own*, Ruth Burgess (Ed.), Wild Goose Publications, 2004

'Homage to young men' – by Alastair McIntosh, chorus by Luke Concannon, from *Love & Revolution*, Alastair McIntosh, Luath Press, 2006. Used by permission of Alastair McIntosh and Luke Concannon

'Receiving (A poem for John)' – by Rachel McCann, from *Down the Track: A Camas Anthology*, Rachel McCann (Ed.), Wild Goose Publications, 2022

'When I have lost my song' – by Elizabeth Baxter was originally written for *Words of Life, 2007*, International Bible Reading Association, Nicola Slee (Ed.). It was also published in *Retreats*. Used by permission of Elizabeth Baxter.

Pieces by Gill Dascombe originally from a series published in the *Methodist Recorder*. Used by permission of Gill Dascombe

'Waiting and hope' – by Thom M Shuman, from *In Love with the Life of Life: Daily Readings for Lent and Holy Week*, Neil Paynter (Ed.), Wild Goose Publications, 2020

'A day in the life … Patrick: children and young people therapist' – by Patrick Bentley, from the Freedom from Torture website (*www.freedomfromtorture.org*), used by permission of Freedom from Torture

'Gary' – by Jan Sutch Pickard, from *Out of Iona: Words from a Crossroads of the World*, Jan Sutch Pickard, Wild Goose Publications, 2003

'Waiting' – by Laura Gisbourne, from *In Love with the Life of Life: Daily Readings for Lent and Holy Week*, Neil Paynter (Ed.), Wild Goose Publications, 2020

'A young man' – by Neil Paynter, adapted from *Light of the World: Daily Readings for Advent*, Peter Millar and Neil Paynter (Eds), Wild Goose Publications, 2009

'David's story'– by Neil Paynter, adapted from *Light of the World: Daily Readings for Advent*, Peter Millar and Neil Paynter (Eds), Wild Goose Publications, 2009

'A child at heart' – from *Coracle,* the magazine of the Iona Community, Neil Paynter (Ed.)

'Burnout' – by Stephen G Wright, from *Coracle,* the magazine of the Iona Community, Neil Paynter (Ed.)

'Cocoa the wonder dog' – by Thom M Shuman, from *Companions on the Journey: A Blessing of Pets and Animals Who Are a Part of Our Lives*, Thom M Shuman, Wild Goose Publications

'Our mutual dependence' – by Iain Whyte, from *Holy Ground: Liturgies and Worship Resources for an Engaged Spirituality,* Helen Boothroyd and Neil Paynter (Eds), Wild Goose Publications, 2005

'A man has died' – first published as 'Another life lost to an asylum system predicated on injustice', by Alison Phipps, *The National*, 16 May 2020. Used by permission of Alison Phipps

'The Buddy Beat', by Tom Chalmers, first published by Scottish Recovery Network (www.scottishrecovery.net)

'Fellowship at the State Hospital' – by Philip Fox, from *Coracle*, the magazine of the Iona Community, Neil Paynter (Ed.)

Other pieces by Neil Paynter adapted from *Down to Earth: Stories and Sketches*, Neil Paynter, Wild Goose Publications, 2009

Wild Goose Publications, the publishing house of the Iona Community established in the Celtic Christian tradition of Saint Columba, produces books, e-books, CDs and digital downloads on:

- holistic spirituality
- social justice
- political and peace issues
- healing
- innovative approaches to worship
- song in worship, including the work of the Wild Goose Resource Group
- material for meditation and reflection

Visit our website at
www.ionabooks.com
for details of all our products and online sales